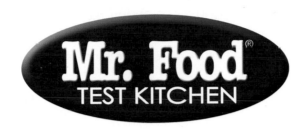

Guilt-Free
Weeknight Favorites

More than 150 New Healthy and Diabetes-Friendly Recipes

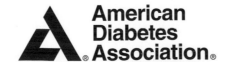

American Diabetes Association

American Diabetes Association team: Director, Book Publishing, Abe Ogden; *Managing Editor,* Greg Guthrie; *Acquisitions Editor,* Victor Van Beuren; *Production Manager,* Melissa Sprott; *Composition Services,* Circle Graphics; *Printer,* Versa Press.

Mr. Food Test Kitchen team: Chief Food Officer, Howard Rosenthal; *Editor,* Jodi Flayman; *Test Kitchen Director,* Patty Rosenthal; *Photography,* Kelly Rusin; *Post Production,* Hal Silverman of Hal Silverman Studio; *Cover and Page Design,* Rachel Johnson.

Printed in the United States of America
1 3 5 7 9 10 8 6 4 2

The suggestions and information contained in this publication are generally consistent with the *Clinical Practice Recommendations* and other policies of the American Diabetes Association, but they do not represent the policy or position of the Association, Cogin, Inc., Ginsburg Enterprises Incorporated, or any of their boards or committees. Reasonable steps have been taken to ensure the accuracy of the information presented. However, the American Diabetes Association cannot ensure the safety or efficacy of any product or service described in this publication. Individuals are advised to consult a physician or other appropriate health care professional before undertaking any diet or exercise program or taking any medication referred to in this publication. Professionals must use and apply their own professional judgment, experience, and training and should not rely solely on the information contained in this publication before prescribing any diet, exercise, or medication. The American Diabetes Association, Cogin, Inc., Ginsburg Enterprises Incorporated—their officers, directors, employees, volunteers, and members—assume no responsibility or liability for personal or other injury, loss, or damage that may result from the suggestions or information in this publication.

∞ The paper in this publication meets the requirements of the ANSI Standard Z39.48-1992 (permanence of paper).

ADA titles may be purchased for business or promotional use or for special sales. To purchase more than 50 copies of this book at a discount, or for custom editions of this book with your logo, contact the American Diabetes Association at the address below, at booksales@diabetes.org, or by calling 703-299-2046.

American Diabetes Association
1701 North Beauregard Street
Alexandria, Virginia 22311

Cogin, Inc.
1770 NW 64 Street, Suite 500
Fort Lauderdale, FL 33309
DOI: 10.2337/9781580405560

Library of Congress Cataloging-in-Publication Data

Mr. Food Test Kitchen's guilt-free weeknight favorites / Mr. Food Test Kitchen.—First edition.
    pages cm
 Includes index.
 ISBN 978-1-58040-556-0 (alk. paper)
 1. Diabetes—Diet therapy—Recipes. I. Mr. Food Test Kitchen (Organization) II. American Diabetes Association.
III. Title. IV. Title: Guilt-free weeknight favorites.

RC662.M73 2015
641.5'6314—dc23

2014042390

Contents

Foreword by Ryan Reed

It may not seem like it, but being a professional race car driver requires being in peak physical condition. And because I have type 1 diabetes, I need to go further than others. This means taking care of me and my diabetes. This means that I have to eat well to manage my diabetes.

There isn't a large selection of healthy foods trackside at most races. So I have learned to be prepared with healthy, nutritious foods at my racing events. But not everyone has a pit crew to provide that kind of support. That's why I'm really glad to see that the American Diabetes Association and the Mr. Food Test Kitchen have teamed up to bring good-tasting, healthy, and nutritious meals to people with diabetes.

Mr. Food Test Kitchen's Guilt-Free Weeknight Favorites takes it all a step further by showing us how to make quick and easy weeknight meals. With my busy schedule and constant traveling to races, I need to know how to make a quick, healthy weeknight meal when my time is at a premium. So I love that I can have some Veggie-Stuffed Pork Chops or Beefy Enchiladas for dinner in less than an hour. And it's even better knowing that the recipe has been tested and ensured to meet the American Diabetes Association's nutrition guidelines. That guarantee gives me the same sense of security as wearing a safety belt.

I was 17 years old when I was diagnosed with type 1 diabetes, and it nearly destroyed my career. I had been racing since I was 4 years old and was living my childhood dream. Now I was being told that I would never race again. But rather than listening to the negativity surrounding me, I decided to pursue my dream no matter what, and that began with finding a new doctor for my diabetes.

Now, I race with a continuous glucose monitor attached to my dashboard. My pit crew is trained to recognize the signs of a medical issue. There's even a target on the leg of my race suit, so the extra man over the wall knows where to give me an injection if it's needed. Having diabetes meant that I had to change my life, but it never meant that I had to give up!

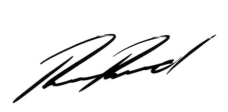

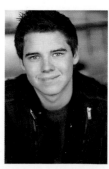

Acknowledgments

Nothing could be more rewarding than being part of a team that strives to make a difference in the lives of others. And like any other big project, developing this cookbook required the dedication and talent of such a team—the staff of the Mr. Food Test Kitchen. So, once again, it's time to recognize all who were committed to creating such an amazing cookbook.

Guilt-Free Weeknight Favorites wouldn't have happened without the watchful eye, organization, and dedication of Jodi Flayman—thank you, as always, for doing us proud. And once again, our deepest thanks go to Patty Rosenthal, who put her heart and soul into every recipe, making sure each one met the strict criteria of both the Mr. Food Test Kitchen and the American Diabetes Association. You are awesome. And every day, as our Test Kitchen Team cooked up a storm, Dave DiCarlo was there to make sure that our kitchen was always kept in tip-top shape.

Once the recipes passed our "triple-tested inspection," it was time for the talented Kelly Rusin to capture each one with her camera and make everything look, as she would say, "quite tasty." We were also fortunate to have the very talented Hal Silverman do his magic during postproduction, so that every image is even more mouthwatering.

When it came to crafting the right words so every recipe is super easy to understand and then proofread them over and over, no one was better than Carol Ginsburg. We thank you. A special thanks also goes to Amy Magro, who helped keep everything running smoothly; Jaime Gross, who was always magically there when we needed her; and Merly Mesa, for keeping us connected with all of you online.

A big thank you goes to Howard Rosenthal, our Chief Food Officer, who not only wears many hats, but also ensures we all carry on the Mr. Food legacy just as Art Ginsburg, our founder, would have wanted. And where would we be without our CEO, Steve Ginsburg, who keeps the company focused as it continues to grow beyond his father's vision? Of course, we'd like to recognize the assistance of our friends at the American Diabetes Association: Abe Ogden, Director, Book Publishing; Greg Guthrie, Managing Editor; and all the talented folks who made sure that all of our recipes complied with their strict standards.

And most of all, thank YOU, our devoted Mr. Food viewers and readers, who have stood by us for more than 30 years, always encouraging us to do our very best. We truly appreciate each and every one of you.

Introduction

Ever find yourself wondering what you're going to make for dinner? And, just as importantly, how you're going to come up with a healthy dinner that fits into your diabetes-friendly meal plan and that the whole family will actually like? We thought so!

The answer is in your hands! Now that you're armed with *Guilt-Free Weeknight Favorites* from the Mr. Food Test Kitchen, there's nothing to worry about! There are more than 150 new, healthy, and diabetes-friendly recipes at your fingertips!

Based on the success of our diabetes-friendly cookbook, *Hello Taste, Goodbye Guilt!*, you asked us for more guilt-free meals, especially ones that are weeknight friendly. So for the last year, our Test Kitchen team, along with the support of the American Diabetes Association (ADA), has been working tirelessly to come up with a cookbook that has just that! And, as expected, you can rest assured knowing that this cookbook follows the strict guidelines of the ADA's dietitians and a whole lot of other folks with fancy-schmancy medical acronyms after their names.

Our goal in this book was not to simply put together a bunch of healthy recipes that taste like "healthy recipes," but rather to come up with recipes that you would never expect to fit your meal plan.

When we say "weeknight favorites," we're talking about dishes like Parmesan-Crusted Chicken (page 93), Simple Southern Sliders (page 109), and Veggie White Lasagna (page 140). We even included a whole chapter of some of our favorite breakfast foods that are dinnertime worthy. Since we can't live on main dishes alone, you can count on there being plenty of tempting go-alongs to round out your meals! Of course, we all know that no weeknight is complete without at least a smidgen of something sweet, which is why we had to include a whole chapter on desserts that we know you're going to fall in love with!

Our promise to you is that these recipes, in addition to getting the stamp of approval from the American Diabetes Association, are so good that you can serve them to your family, friends, or really anyone who appreciates great-tasting food. They'll never know that they're diabetes friendly.

Alright—enough chit-chat from us. It's time to get cooking and start tasting all of the "OOH IT'S SO GOOD!!®"

Sugar: Good or Bad?

There seem to be a lot of questions about the role sugar plays in diabetes, so we dug a little deeper. Some folks insist that if you eat too much sugar, you will get type 1 diabetes, but consuming sugar has nothing to do with developing that form of the disease. It is caused by genetics and other unknown factors that trigger the disease. With type 2 diabetes, however, being overweight is a key risk for developing the disease, and a lot of excess calories come from sugar (especially sugary beverages like soda) in the diet.

In the past, it was thought that if you had diabetes, you couldn't eat sugar at all. Years of research have shown that even though sugar can raise your blood glucose levels, it's more important to watch the total amount of carbohydrates you consume. These days, experts agree that you can include sugar and other carbohydrate-containing foods in your meal plan—as long as you do so in moderation—and still keep your blood glucose levels in your target range.

This doesn't mean that you can eat all the sugar you want. The key is to use sugar in moderation in what you are making and then to remember to eat small serving sizes, so you can keep your carbohydrates in check.

We suggest that you focus on eating a healthy, well-balanced diet. If your meal plan allows you the additional carbs, then by all means, go ahead and satisfy your sweet tooth.

How to Read a Nutrition Facts Label

One of the most important things you can do to help manage your diabetes and to eat healthy is to learn how to not only read a nutrition label, but to understand it, too. It's really quite simple once you learn a few basic tips.

- **Serving Size:** This is the standard or recommended portion you are supposed to eat of this item. The key word is "recommended." You may find that your serving size fluctuates quite a bit depending upon how small or large your appetite is. Please be realistic here and remember that portion control is a huge factor in diabetes management.

- **Servings per Container:** This number will vary based on the serving size. Each food group has a recommended serving size. The bigger the serving size, the fewer servings per container. So, for example, if you eat an entire jumbo bag of potato chips in one sitting, remember that the entire bag is not considered one serving!

- **The Basics:** To best help manage our diets, it is most important to know the basic nutritional components: fat, saturated fat, cholesterol, sodium, carbohydrate, and a few vitamins contained in almost all foods. That's why these are listed not only in grams or milligrams, but also as a percentage of an average person's daily allotment, based on a daily 2,000-calorie (or sometimes also a 2,500-calorie) diet. Your own "Daily Values" for these items may be higher or lower, depending on your level of activity and your personal needs.

Nutrition Facts

Serving Size 1 cup (53g/1.9 oz)
Servings Per Container About 8

Amount Per Serving

Calories 190	**Calories from Fat** 25

	% Daily Value**
Total Fat 3g*	**5%**
Saturated Fat 0g	**0%**
Trans Fat 0g	
Cholesterol 0mg	**0%**
Sodium 95mg	**4%**
Potassium 300mg	**9%**
Total Carbohydrate 36g	**12%**
Dietary Fiber 8g	**32%**
Soluble Fiber 3g	
Sugars 13g	
Protein 9g	**14%**

Vitamin A 0%	•	Vitamin C 0%
Calcium 4%	•	Iron 10%
Phosphorus 10%	•	Magnesium 10%
Copper 8%		

*Amount in Cereal. One half cup of fat free milk contributes an additional 40 calories, 65mg sodium, 6g total carbohydrates (6g sugars), and 4g protein.
**Percent Daily Values are based on a 2,000 calorie diet. Your Daily Values may be higher or lower depending on your calorie needs.

		Calories:	2,000	2,500
Total Fat	Less than		65g	80g
Sat Fat	Less than		20g	25g
Cholesterol	Less than		300mg	300mg
Sodium	Less than		2,400mg	2,400mg
Potassium			3,500mg	3,500mg
Total Carbohydrate			300g	375g
Dietary Fiber			25g	30g

Calories per gram:
Fat 9 • Carbohydrate 4 • Protein 4

- **Minerals and Vitamins:** Only two vitamins, A and C, and two minerals, calcium and iron, are required to be listed on food labels. Food companies often voluntarily list others. If they do, make that information work for you!

Some labels also list the approximate number of calories in a gram of fat, carbohydrate, and protein. When available, these numbers can be useful as you create your meal plans.

You shouldn't have to look too hard for nutrition information, because the FDA regulates the size of the labels. The FDA also has strict guidelines regarding the information that is contained in these labels. This means that we can count on them being large and clear enough to be easily read and understood.

As always, if you'd like further information on better understanding how these nutrition labels impact your dietary intake, or how to shape your own meal plan, the best place to start is with your physician, a registered dietitian, or a health-care professional.

When calculating nutrition, we use the following guidelines:

- When cooking pasta, we don't add salt to the water.

- We use regular pasta when testing recipes to be sure they meet nutritional guidelines, but you can substitute whole-grain pasta if you're looking to reduce carbs and increase fiber, or even try mixing half and half.

- We use medium-sized fruits and vegetables unless otherwise specified.

- We use 95% extra-lean ground beef unless otherwise specified.

- We use well-trimmed meat.

- We use thin-sliced chicken cutlets whenever possible.

- We use light, trans-fat-free, tub-style margarine unless otherwise specified.

- We discard any unused breading or marinade, and these amounts are not figured in our nutritional calculations.

- Nutritional information is based on the serving size shown. Make sure you keep this in mind while you are dishing up a recipe.

All-Important Portion Control

Is it really such a big deal if you eat a smidgen more than what your meal plan calls for? You might think that an extra bite or two of something won't really affect anything, but it does make a difference! Those extra calories add up, making it that much harder to control diabetes. That's where portion control comes in.

How do you measure up?

We certainly don't expect anyone to run around with a food scale, so here are a few easy ways you can measure your foods:

- Try this with fruits and veggies. In the supermarket produce section, pick up small, medium, and large pieces of fruit and veggies in your hands and guesstimate their weight, then weigh them on the store's scale. How close are you? After doing this a few times, you'll be able to fairly accurately guess the weight of most fruit and veggies. That's the start of portion control!

- Measure it before serving it. When it comes to adding milk to your cereal, do you really measure and add exactly the one cup that is suggested? No way! But here is what we recommend. Simply measure one cup of any liquid in a measuring cup, then pour the liquid into one of your everyday drinking glasses. Mark or memorize where the liquid comes up to. It's so easy! This method can actually be applied to just about anything, from how much cereal to put in your bowl to how much oil you use to coat your skillet. It's always best to be aware of exactly what you're taking in.

- When you eat out, portion control can get a bit tricky. If you go to a restaurant that serves large portions, split your meal with someone at the table, or better yet, when your meal arrives, set aside half to bring home for lunch or dinner the next day. It will truly make a difference.

After practicing these tips, you'll be able to tell the sizes of your portions just by looking at them. Just be sure to practice guesstimating portion sizes whenever you're in the grocery store to keep your internal food scale "calibrated." It's really not that hard, and you can even turn it into a game! The winner? You, of course!

Here's a visual tool that references everyday objects to help you compare food portions:

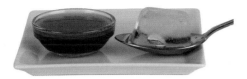
2 tablespoons salad dressing = ice cube

3 ounces meat = deck of cards

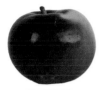
medium apple = tennis ball

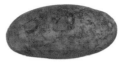
medium potato = computer mouse

medium onion = baseball

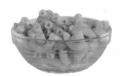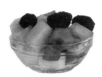
1 cup cut fruit = medium orange

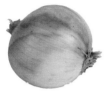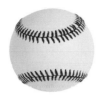
1 ounce meat = matchbox

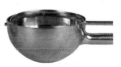
1/2 cup cooked pasta = ice cream scoop

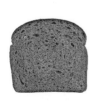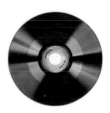
1 ounce bread = CD or DVD

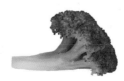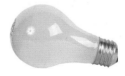
1 cup broccoli = light bulb

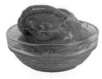
2 tablespoons peanut butter = golf ball

1 ounce cheese = domino

Notes

Breakfast Anytime

Veggie-Packed Grits 'n' Eggs

Serves 4, 1 egg and about 1 cup grits and vegetables per serving

4	cups water
1	cup quick-cooking grits
1/4	cup diced onion
1/4	cup diced red bell pepper
1/2	teaspoon salt
1/4	teaspoon black pepper
2	cups fresh baby spinach, roughly chopped
4	eggs
1/4	cup (1 ounce) shredded reduced-fat Parmesan cheese

1 In a medium saucepan over high heat, boil water. Add grits, stirring constantly. Add onion, red bell pepper, salt, and pepper, and return to a boil; reduce heat to medium. Cook 5 to 7 minutes, or until water is absorbed and mixture is thickened, stirring occasionally. Add spinach, stirring until wilted. Cover and keep warm.

2 Meanwhile, in a nonstick skillet, cook eggs sunny-side up, in batches.

3 Divide grits evenly on 4 serving plates and top each with a fried egg. Sprinkle with cheese and serve immediately.

Good for You!
Did you know that by adding the veggies to the grits we added lots of good-for-you vitamins, minerals, and fiber that our body needs?

Choices/Exchanges, 2 starch, 1 nonstarchy vegetable, 1 medium-fat protein

Calories 250, Calories From Fat 60, **Total Fat** 7.0g, Saturated Fat 2.5g, Trans Fat 0.0g, **Cholesterol** 215mg, **Sodium** 460mg, **Potassium** 240mg, **Total Carbohydrates** 34g, Fiber 1g, Sugar 2g, **Protein** 12g, **Phosphorus** 175mg

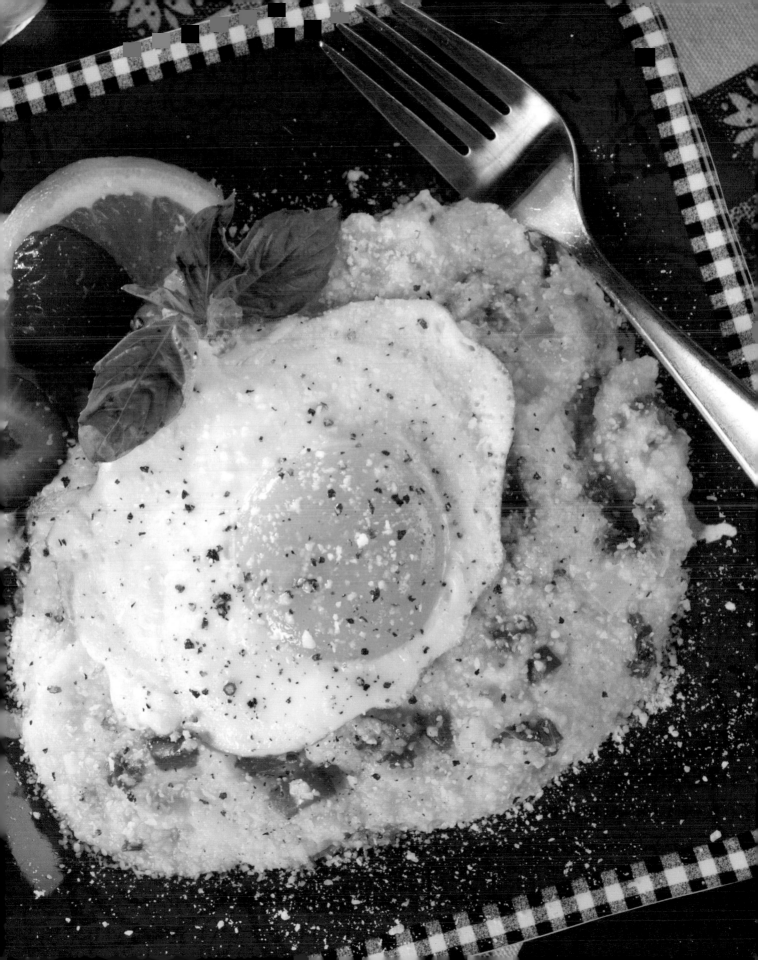

Baked Egg Casserole

Serves 6, 1 piece per serving

4	slices reduced-calorie whole-grain bread, cubed
1-1/2	cups liquid egg substitute
1	cup fat-free evaporated milk
1	cup crumbled reduced-fat feta cheese, divided
1/2	teaspoon dried oregano
3/4	teaspoon onion powder
3	scallions, thinly sliced
2	tablespoons sliced black olives

1 Preheat oven to 325°F. Coat a 9-inch pie plate with cooking spray. Arrange bread cubes in pie plate.

2 In a medium bowl, combine liquid egg, evaporated milk, 1/2 cup cheese, oregano, onion powder, scallions, and black olives.

3 Pour egg mixture over bread cubes, gently pushing cubes down into liquid. Let stand 5 minutes and push cubes into liquid again, making sure the bread is well coated. Sprinkle with remaining cheese.

4 Cover and bake 15 minutes. Remove cover and bake 10 to 15 additional minutes, or until golden and a knife inserted in center comes out clean. Cut into 6 pieces and serve immediately.

Good for You!

A good way to add flavor to recipes, but not lots of sodium, is to mix in small amounts of items like olives or pickles. Here the olives lend the saltiness we crave but with less added sodium.

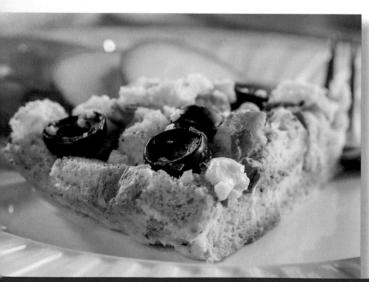

Choices/Exchanges, 1 carbohydrate, 2 lean protein

Calories 140, Calories From Fat 35, **Total Fat** 4.0g, Saturated Fat 1.0g, Trans Fat 0.0g, **Cholesterol** 5mg, **Sodium** 300mg, **Potassium** 390mg, **Total Carbohydrates** 13g, Fiber 2g, Sugar 6g, **Protein** 13g, **Phosphorus** 185mg

Roasted Veggie Frittata

Serves 8, 1 piece per serving

1	red bell pepper, cut into strips
1	onion, thinly sliced
1	cup mushrooms, sliced
2	teaspoons olive oil
1/4	teaspoon salt
1/4	teaspoon black pepper
1	teaspoon Italian seasoning
1/2	cup fresh baby spinach
1/4	cup goat cheese crumbles
3	cups liquid egg whites

1 Preheat oven to 400°F. Coat a rimmed baking sheet and a 9 × 13-inch baking dish with cooking spray. Set aside.

2 In a large bowl, toss bell pepper, onion, and mushrooms with olive oil, salt, pepper, and Italian seasoning. Spread evenly onto baking sheet.

3 Roast 18 to 20 minutes, or until vegetables are tender. Remove from oven and reduce oven to 325°F.

4 Return vegetables to bowl and toss with spinach. Spread in prepared baking dish and sprinkle with goat cheese. Pour egg whites evenly over top.

5 Bake 30 to 35 minutes, or until a knife inserted in center comes out clean. Let stand 5 minutes; cut into 8 pieces and serve.

Test Kitchen. Mr. Food Hints & Tips

We found that roasting vegetables brings out their natural sweet flavors, which give this dish tons of taste. Also, compared with traditional cheeses, goat cheese is lower in fat, calories, and cholesterol, and a little goes a long way. So dig in without any guilt.

Choices/Exchanges, 1 nonstarchy vegetable, 1 lean protein, 1/2 fat

Calories 90, Calories From Fat 25, **Total Fat** 3.0g, Saturated Fat 1.0g, Trans Fat 0.0g, **Cholesterol** <5mg, **Sodium** 260mg, **Potassium** 260mg, **Total Carbohydrates** 4g, Fiber <1g, Sugar 2g, **Protein** 12g, **Phosphorus** 35mg

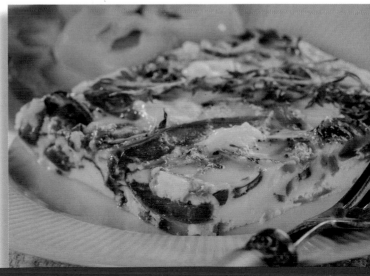

Cantina Egg Burrito

Serves 4, 1 burrito per serving

1/2	cup canned black beans, rinsed and drained
2/3	cup medium salsa, divided
1/2	teaspoon cumin
4	eggs
2	tablespoons fat-free milk
1/8	teaspoon salt
1/4	teaspoon black pepper
1	tomato, diced
1/2	cup (2 ounces) shredded fat-free sharp Cheddar cheese
1/4	cup reduced-fat sour cream
2	tablespoons chopped fresh cilantro

1 In a small saucepan, coarsely mash the black beans. Add 1/3 cup salsa and cumin; heat over low heat until heated through. Cover and keep warm.

2 In a medium bowl, whisk eggs, milk, salt, and pepper.

3 Coat a medium skillet with cooking spray and heat over medium heat. Pour 1/4 cup egg mixture into pan. Tilt pan to spread egg mixture to completely cover bottom with a thin layer. Cook 1-1/2 to 2 minutes, or until lightly browned on bottom. Loosen edges with spatula and carefully slide out onto a serving plate, browned side down. (It will look like a tortilla.) Repeat with the rest of the egg mixture.

4 Spread 1/4 of the bean mixture down the center of a "tortilla." Top with 1/4 of the tomato and 1/4 of the cheese. Roll up loosely. Keep warm while preparing and assembling remaining burritos. Top evenly with sour cream and remaining salsa, garnish with cilantro, and serve.

Good for You!
Draining and rinsing canned beans helps remove excess sodium and starch, while improving their flavor.

Choices/Exchanges, 1/2 starch, 1 nonstarchy vegetable, 1 medium-fat protein

Calories 150, Calories From Fat 50, **Total Fat** 6.0g, Saturated Fat 2.0g, Trans Fat 0.0g, **Cholesterol** 215mg, **Sodium** 480mg, **Potassium** 340mg, **Total Carbohydrates** 11g, Fiber 3g, Sugar 4g, **Protein** 14g, **Phosphorus** 155mg

Meat Lover's Breakfast Cups

Serves 6, 1 cup per serving

1-1/4 cups frozen shredded hash brown potatoes, thawed
1 teaspoon canola oil
2 tablespoons finely chopped onion
1 garlic clove, minced
2 frozen turkey sausage patties, thawed and diced
1 tablespoon fat-free sour cream
1 cup liquid egg substitute
1/4 teaspoon salt
1/8 teaspoon black pepper
2 tablespoons turkey bacon pieces
2 tablespoons shredded Monterey Jack cheese

1 Preheat oven to 400°F. Coat a 6-cup muffin tin with cooking spray. Evenly divide hash browns into bottom and up sides of each muffin cup, pressing firmly.

2 In a large skillet over medium heat, sauté onion in oil until tender. Add garlic and sausage; cook 1 more minute. Remove from heat; stir in sour cream.

3 In a medium bowl, beat liquid egg with salt and pepper, then pour evenly into potato-lined muffin cups. Top with sausage mixture and sprinkle with bacon and cheese.

4 Bake 15 to 18 minutes, or until eggs are set. Serve immediately.

Serving Suggestion
Serve these with some fresh fruit, and you have a breakfast or brunch that looks very fancy.

Choices/Exchanges, 1/2 carbohydrate, 1 lean protein, 1/2 fat

Calories 110, Calories From Fat 45, **Total Fat** 5.0g, Saturated Fat 1.5g, Trans Fat 0.0g, **Cholesterol** 60mg, **Sodium** 340mg, **Potassium** 150mg, **Total Carbohydrates** 9g, Fiber <1g, Sugar <1g, **Protein** 8g, **Phosphorus** 50mg

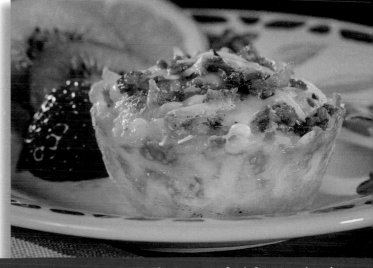

Country Breakfast in a Mug

Serves 1

1   egg, beaten
1   tablespoon water
1   (1-ounce) slice reduced-sodium deli ham, chopped
1/4   cup frozen chopped broccoli, thawed and squeezed dry
1/8   teaspoon salt (optional)
1/8   teaspoon black pepper
1   tablespoon shredded reduced-fat sharp Cheddar cheese

1 Coat an 8-ounce microwaveable mug with cooking spray. Add egg, water, ham, and broccoli; beat with a fork until blended.

2 Microwave on high 30 seconds; stir. Microwave 30 to 45 seconds longer, or until egg is almost set.

3 Season with salt, if desired, and pepper. Top with cheese and serve.

Good for You!
This recipe is an excellent source of protein because of the egg, the ham, and the cheese. It's also the kind of breakfast that keeps your stomach from growling until lunch.

Choices/Exchanges, 2 lean protein, 1/2 fat

Calories 130, Calories From Fat 50, **Total Fat** 6.0g, Saturated Fat 1.5g, Trans Fat 0.0g, **Cholesterol** 225mg, **Sodium** 380mg, **Potassium** 160mg, **Total Carbohydrates** 4g, Fiber 1g, Sugar 2g, **Protein** 15g, **Phosphorus** 115mg

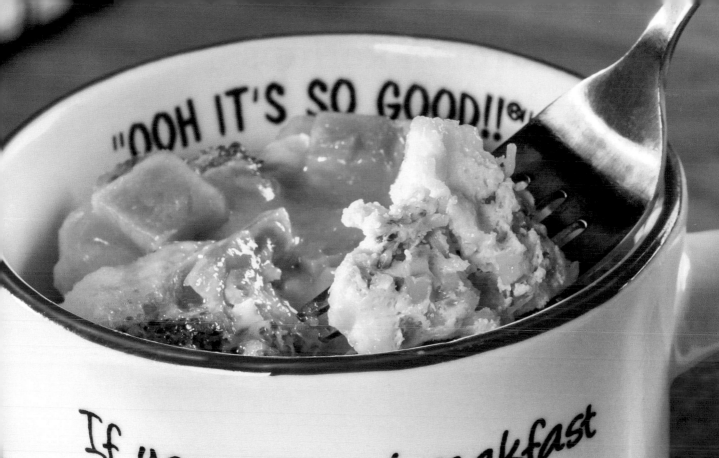

"OOH IT'S SO GOOD!!®"

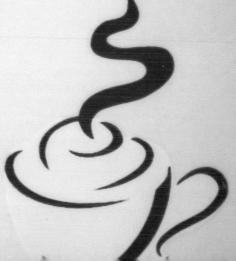

If you want breakfast in bed, sleep in the kitchen !

Smoked Salmon Rollups

Serves 4, 1 rollup per serving

1/3	cup fat-free vegetable cream cheese
4	(7-inch) whole-wheat tortillas
4	ounces thinly sliced smoked salmon, cut into strips
1	small cucumber, very thinly sliced
1	tomato, very thinly sliced

1 Spread cream cheese evenly over tortillas. Divide salmon evenly over bottom half of each tortilla. Layer cucumber and tomato slices over salmon.

2 Starting from the bottom, roll up tortillas. Cut in half and serve.

Just a Thought
You can make these a day ahead of time and simply wrap them snugly in wax paper. That way they not only stay fresh, they are ready and waiting for you for the perfect on-the-go breakfast or snack.

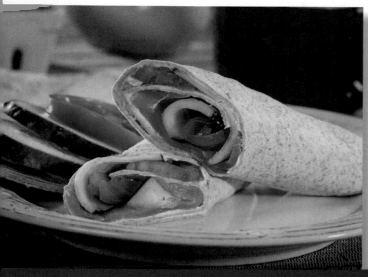

Choices/Exchanges, 1 starch, 1/2 carbohydrate, 1 lean protein, 1/2 fat

Calories 190, Calories From Fat 45, **Total Fat** 5.0g, Saturated Fat 1.5g, Trans Fat 0.0g, **Cholesterol** 10mg, **Sodium** 600mg, **Potassium** 270mg, **Total Carbohydrates** 24g, Fiber 4g, Sugar 2g, **Protein** 12g, **Phosphorus** 155mg

Bacon Lover's Pancakes

Serves 6, 4 silver-dollar pancakes per serving

4	slices lower-sodium turkey bacon
1-1/2	cups dry pancake mix
1/2	cup low-fat milk
1/2	cup fat-free plain yogurt
1/2	cup liquid egg substitute
	Sugar-free maple syrup for drizzling (optional)

1 In a large skillet over medium-low heat, cook bacon until crisp; drain and coarsely chop.

2 In a large bowl, combine pancake mix, milk, yogurt, and liquid egg; mix until well combined.

3 Coat a griddle or large skillet with cooking spray. Over medium heat, pour silver dollar-sized amounts of pancake batter onto griddle and sprinkle evenly with chopped bacon. Cook 2 to 3 minutes, or until bubbles begin to form; then turn over and cook 1 to 2 additional minutes, or until golden. Continue to cook in batches until all of the batter is used.

4 Drizzle with warmed syrup, if desired, and serve.

Good for You!
If you want to make these even healthier, you can use whole-wheat pancake mix, which will provide you with even more fiber and iron.

Choices/Exchanges, 1 1/2 starch, 1 lean protein

Calories 160, Calories From Fat 25, **Total Fat** 2.5g, Saturated Fat 1.0g, Trans Fat 0.0g, **Cholesterol** 10mg, **Sodium** 480mg, **Potassium** 190mg, **Total Carbohydrates** 23g, Fiber 2g, Sugar 2g, **Protein** 8g, **Phosphorus** 220mg

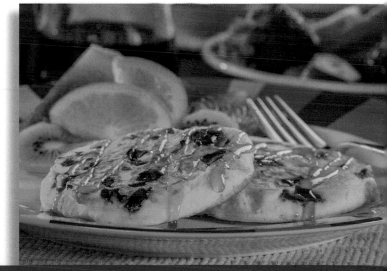

Chocolate Chip Waffles

Serves 6, 1 waffle per serving

1-1/2	cups all-purpose flour
1	cup quick-cooking oats
3	teaspoons baking powder
1/2	teaspoon cinnamon
1/4	teaspoon salt (optional)
1-1/2	cups fat-free milk
1/2	cup liquid egg substitute, lightly beaten
4	tablespoons (1/4 cup) light, trans-fat-free margarine, melted
2	tablespoons brown sugar
2	tablespoons mini chocolate chips

1 Preheat electric or stovetop waffle iron. Coat with cooking spray.

2 In a large bowl, combine flour, oats, baking powder, cinnamon, and salt, if desired; set aside.

3 In a small bowl, whisk the milk, liquid egg, margarine, and brown sugar. Add to flour mixture and stir until blended. Stir in chocolate chips.

4 Pour 1/3 to 1/2 cup batter evenly onto waffle iron, but not all the way to the edges, as batter will spread when waffle iron is closed. Cook about 1-1/2 minutes, or until golden. Carefully remove waffle from waffle iron with a fork. Repeat with remaining batter, spraying waffle iron with cooking spray between each waffle.

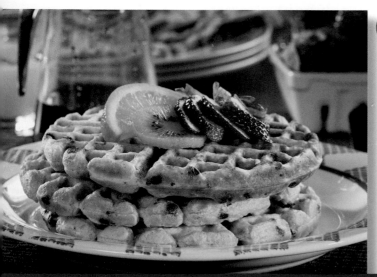

Test Kitchen. Mr. Food Hints & Tips

We use mini chocolate chips as a way to ensure you have chocolate in every bite without adding lots of extra carbs. You'll definitely feel like you're indulging with this treat.

Choices/Exchanges, 3 carbohydrate, 1 lean protein

Calories 260, Calories From Fat 45, **Total Fat** 5.0g, Saturated Fat 1.5g, Trans Fat 0.0g, **Cholesterol** 0mg, **Sodium** 380mg, **Potassium** 230mg, **Total Carbohydrates** 44g, Fiber 2g, Sugar 8g, **Protein** 10g, **Phosphorus** 220mg

Southern Pecan Oatmeal

Serves 6, 3/4 cup per serving

3-1/2	cups water
2	tablespoons honey
1/2	teaspoon cinnamon
1/2	teaspoon salt (optional)
2	cups quick-cooking steel-cut oats
1/2	cup chopped pecans, divided
1/4	cup sugar-free caramel topping, warmed

1 In a 3-quart saucepan over high heat, bring water, honey, cinnamon, and salt, if desired, to a boil. Stir in oats; return to boil. Reduce heat to medium; cook 5 to 7 minutes, or until most of the liquid is absorbed, stirring occasionally.

2 Remove from heat and stir in 1/3 cup pecans. Divide evenly into 6 bowls, sprinkle with remaining pecans, drizzle with warm caramel topping, and serve immediately.

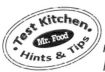

Although you could use regular oatmeal in this recipe, we recommend the steel-cut variety. It is digested more slowly and has a lower glycemic index, which helps keep your blood glucose in check.

Choices/Exchanges, 1 starch, 1 carbohydrate, 1 1/2 fat

Calories 220, Calories From Fat 80, **Total Fat** 9.0g, Saturated Fat 1.0g, Trans Fat 0.0g, **Cholesterol** 0mg, **Sodium** 30mg, **Potassium** 150mg, **Total Carbohydrates** 33g, Fiber 4g, Sugar 6g, **Protein** 4g, **Phosphorus** 145mg

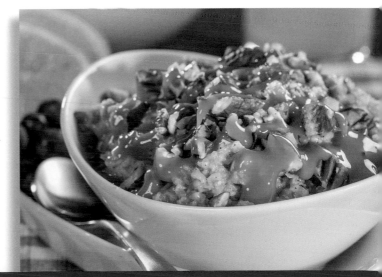

Peach Melba Waffle Soufflés

Serves 5, 1 soufflé per serving

4   frozen whole-wheat waffles, lightly toasted and cut into bite-sized pieces

1   cup fresh or frozen diced peaches, thawed if frozen

1/2   cup sugar-free red raspberry preserves

1/2   cup fat-free milk

3   eggs

3   tablespoons light pancake syrup

1   tablespoon light, trans-fat-free margarine, melted

1   teaspoon vanilla extract

1   teaspoon confectioners' sugar

1 Preheat oven to 325°F. Coat 5 ramekins or custard cups with cooking spray; set aside.

2 In a large bowl, combine waffle pieces, peaches, and raspberry preserves; divide evenly between ramekins.

3 In the same bowl, whisk together milk, eggs, syrup, margarine, and vanilla. Pour over waffle mixture, dividing evenly; press down lightly with a spoon. Place ramekins on a baking sheet.

4 Bake 40 to 45 minutes, or until puffed, and a knife inserted in center of each comes out clean. Cool on a wire rack 5 minutes. Sprinkle with confectioners' sugar and serve warm.

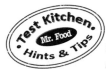

If you don't have individual ramekins or if you want to make one big casserole dish of this, you can use a 1-1/2 quart casserole dish, but bake it 55 to 60 minutes to cook it through.

Choices/Exchanges, 1 1/2 carbohydrate, 1 lean protein

Calories 150, Calories From Fat 40, **Total Fat** 4.5g, Saturated Fat 1.0g, Trans Fat 0.0g, **Cholesterol** 125mg, **Sodium** 280mg, **Potassium** 170mg, **Total Carbohydrates** 22g, Fiber 3g, Sugar 10g, **Protein** 7g, **Phosphorus** 110mg

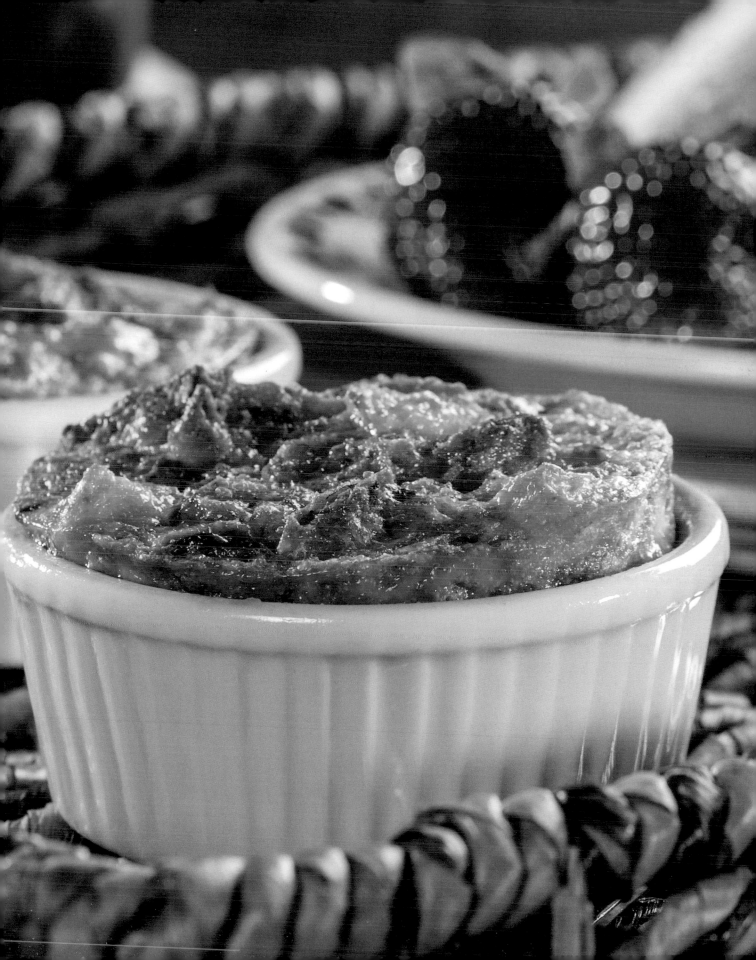

Strawberry Breakfast Bruschetta

Serves 10, 1 slice per serving

10	(1/2-inch) slices French bread
	Cooking spray
3/4	cup fat-free vanilla Greek yogurt
3	teaspoons granulated Splenda
1/2	teaspoon vanilla extract
1-1/2	cups sliced fresh strawberries
1/4	cup chopped pecans
2	teaspoons confectioners' sugar

1 Preheat broiler. Place bread slices on a baking sheet and lightly coat with cooking spray. Broil 1 to 2 minutes, or until lightly browned.

2 In a small bowl, combine yogurt, Splenda, and vanilla. Spread over bread slices.

3 Top evenly with strawberries and pecans, and dust with confectioners' sugar. Serve immediately.

Did You Know?

Are you are thinking: bruschetta for breakfast? Why not? The word "bruschetta" is based on the translation of "bread being toasted over hot coals." We think our new version is very tasty. Let us know what you think on Facebook.

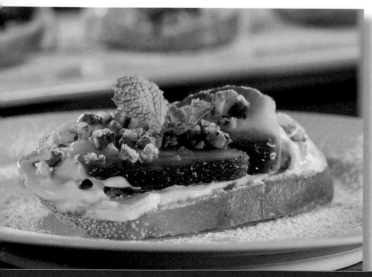

Choices/Exchanges, 1 carbohydrate, 1/2 fat

Calories 115, Calories From Fat 20, **Total Fat** 2.5g, Saturated Fat 0.3g, Trans Fat 0g, **Cholesterol** 0mg, **Sodium** 135mg, **Potassium** 100mg, **Total Carbohydrates** 19g, Fiber 1g, Sugar 4g, **Protein** 5g, **Phosphorus** 60mg

Lemon Blueberry Coffee Cake

Serves 8, 1 slice per serving

1-1/4	cups all-purpose flour, plus extra for dusting
1/2	cup granulated Splenda
1/2	teaspoon baking powder
1/2	teaspoon baking soda
1/4	teaspoon salt
1/4	teaspoon cinnamon
1	egg, beaten
2/3	cup fat-free plain yogurt
2	tablespoons canola oil
1/2	teaspoon vanilla extract
1	cup fresh blueberries
1	tablespoon grated lemon zest

1 Preheat oven to 350°F. Coat a 9-inch cake pan with cooking spray and dust lightly with flour.

2 In a large bowl, stir together 1-1/4 cups flour, Splenda, baking powder, baking soda, salt, and cinnamon; set aside.

3 In a small bowl, combine egg, yogurt, oil, and vanilla.

4 Make a well in center of flour mixture and add egg mixture into the well. Stir just until moistened, with a few lumps remaining. Gently stir in blueberries and lemon zest. Spread batter into prepared pan.

5 Bake 25 to 30 minutes, or until toothpick inserted in center comes out clean. Cut into 8 slices and serve warm.

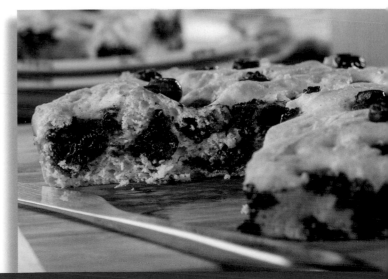

Choices/Exchanges, 1 1/2 carbohydrate, 1 fat

Calories 140, Calories From Fat 40, Total Fat 4.5g, Saturated Fat 0.5g, Trans Fat 0.0g, Cholesterol 30mg, Sodium 210mg, Potassium 95mg, Total Carbohydrates 21g, Fiber 1g, Sugar 2g, Protein 4g, Phosphorus 40mg

Anytime Scones

Serves 12, 1 scone per serving

1-1/2	cups plus 1 tablespoon all-purpose flour, divided
1/2	teaspoon baking soda
1/4	teaspoon salt
2	tablespoons plus 2 teaspoons granulated Splenda, divided
1	teaspoon cream of tartar
3	tablespoons light, trans-fat-free margarine, chilled and cut into pieces
1	cup shredded zucchini
1/3	cup mini chocolate chips
3/4	cup fat-free buttermilk

1 Preheat oven to 375°F. Coat a baking sheet with cooking spray.

2 In a large bowl, combine 1-1/2 cups flour, baking soda, salt, 2 tablespoons Splenda, and cream of tartar. Cut in margarine with a pastry blender or 2 forks, until mixture resembles coarse meal. Stir in zucchini and chocolate chips, tossing well. Add buttermilk, stirring just until dry ingredients are moistened.

3 Sprinkle remaining flour evenly over work surface. Turn dough out onto floured surface; knead 4 or 5 times. Divide dough into 2 portions. Pat each portion into a 5-inch circle on prepared baking sheet. Score each circle into 6 wedges. Sprinkle each circle evenly with remaining Splenda.

4 Bake 25 to 30 minutes, or until golden and center is dry. Cool slightly, then separate into wedges.

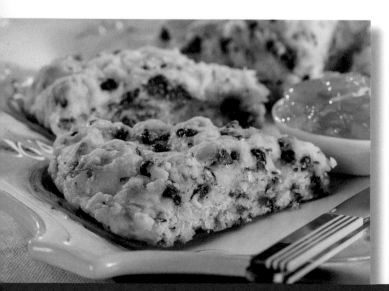

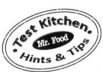

We found that scoring the dough allows us to bake it as a whole so it stays moist, but also allows us to easily break the circles into individual wedges after baking.

Choices/Exchanges, 1 carbohydrate, 1/2 fat

Calories 100, Calories From Fat 25, **Total Fat** 2.5g, Saturated Fat 1.0g, Trans Fat 0.0g, **Cholesterol** 0mg, **Sodium** 130mg, **Potassium** 80mg, **Total Carbohydrates** 17g, Fiber <1g, Sugar 0g, **Protein** 2g, **Phosphorus** 20mg

Watermelon Patch Smoothie

Serves 4, 1 cup per serving

4 cups watermelon chunks
2/3 cup fat-free vanilla Greek yogurt
1 tablespoon honey
1 tablespoon chopped mint, plus extra for garnish
1 cup ice cubes

1 Combine all ingredients in a blender and blend until smooth. Garnish with extra mint and serve immediately.

Just a Thought

This is a great breakfast to take on the go. Just pour it into your favorite travel mug or water bottle, and you can "eat" your breakfast on the way to school or work.

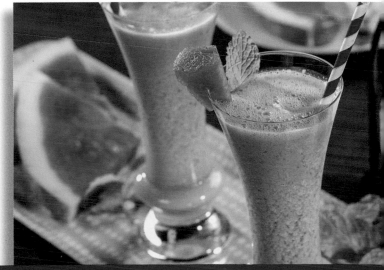

Choices/Exchanges, 1 carbohydrate

Calories 80, Calories From Fat 0, **Total Fat** 0.0g, Saturated Fat 0.0g, Trans Fat 0.0g, **Cholesterol** <5g, **Sodium** 15mg, **Potassium** 220mg, **Total Carbohydrates** 17g, Fiber <1g, Sugar 15g, **Protein** 5g, **Phosphorus** 15mg

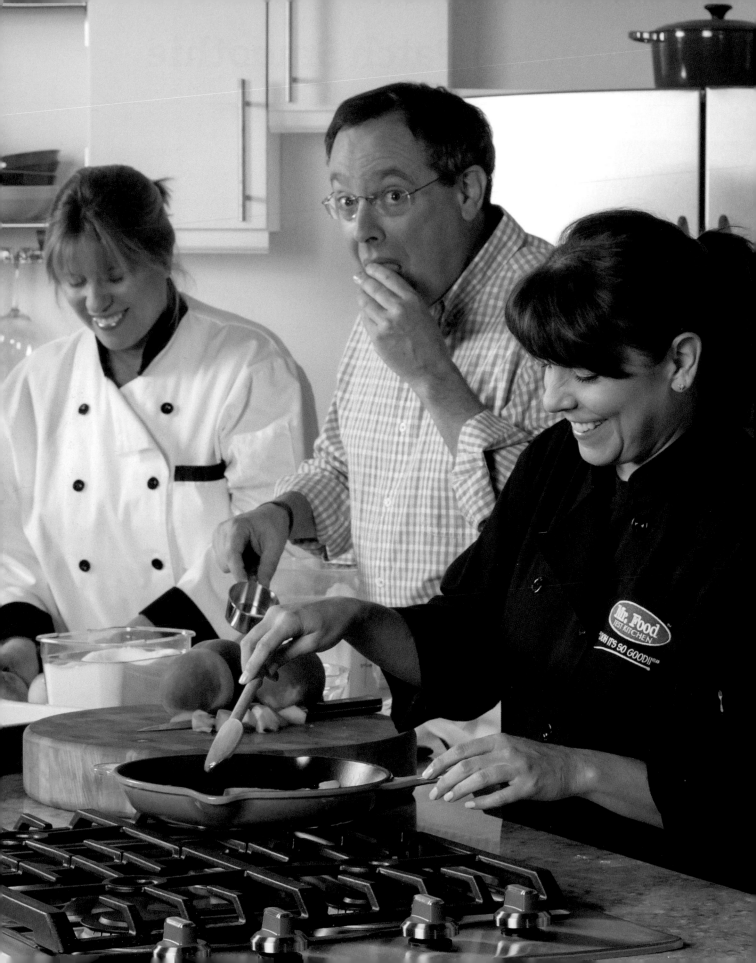

Watermelon Patch Smoothie

Serves 4, 1 cup per serving

4	cups watermelon chunks
2/3	cup fat-free vanilla Greek yogurt
1	tablespoon honey
1	tablespoon chopped mint, plus extra for garnish
1	cup ice cubes

1 Combine all ingredients in a blender and blend until smooth. Garnish with extra mint and serve immediately.

Just a Thought
This is a great breakfast to take on the go. Just pour it into your favorite travel mug or water bottle, and you can "eat" your breakfast on the way to school or work.

Choices/Exchanges, 1 carbohydrate

Calories 80, Calories From Fat 0, **Total Fat** 0.0g, Saturated Fat 0.0g, Trans Fat 0.0g, **Cholesterol** <5g, **Sodium** 15mg, **Potassium** 220mg, **Total Carbohydrates** 17g, Fiber <1g, Sugar 15g, **Protein** 5g, **Phosphorus** 15mg

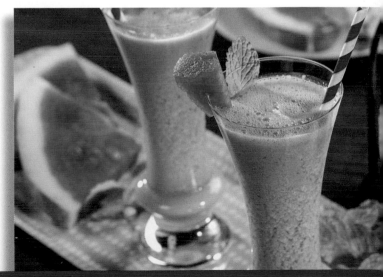

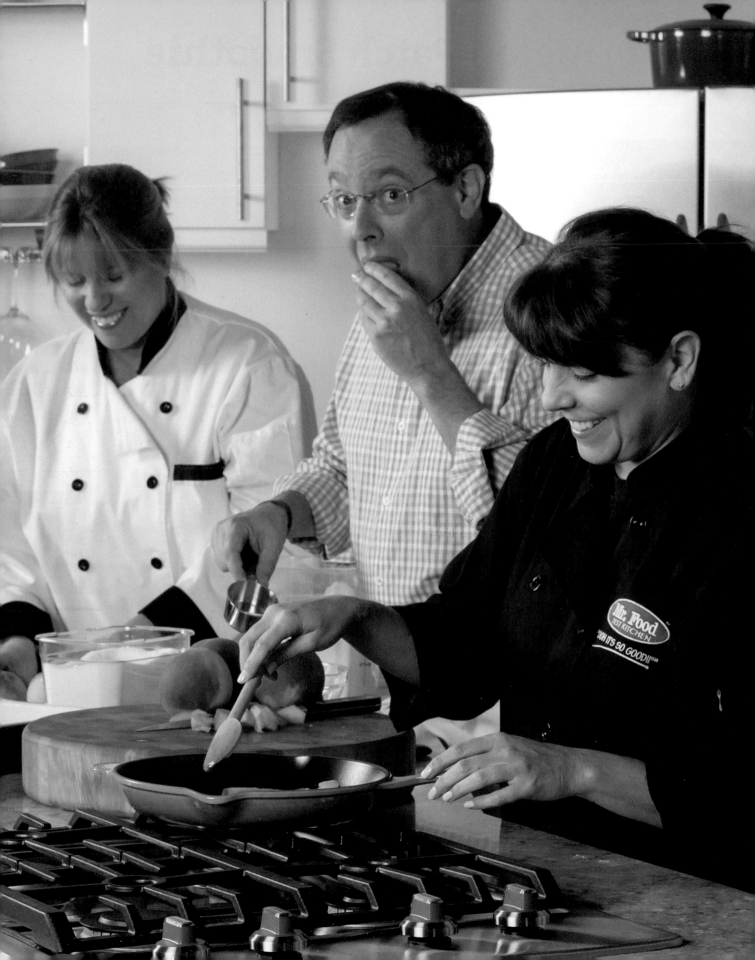

Simply Appetizers

Mini Salmon Cakes

Serves 12, 1 patty per serving

1 pound skinless salmon fillets, cut into chunks
1 slice fresh white bread, torn up
2 scallions, sliced
1 tablespoon lemon juice
1/2 teaspoon garlic powder
1/4 teaspoon salt
1/4 teaspoon black pepper

1 Place all ingredients in a food processor and pulse until coarsely chopped and well combined. Form mixture into 12 mini patties.

2 Coat a skillet or grill pan with cooking spray. Over medium-high heat, cook patties 3 to 4 minutes per side, or until cooked through.

Serving Suggestion

For a quick and easy dipping sauce, mix together 1/3 cup plain low-fat Greek yogurt, 1/3 cup light mayonnaise, 1/2 teaspoon garlic powder, 1/8 teaspoon pepper, and 1 tablespoon capers. It sure doesn't get any easier than this.

Choices/Exchanges, 1 lean protein, 1/2 fat

Calories 80, Calories From Fat 35, **Total Fat** 4.0g, Saturated Fat 1.0g, Trans Fat 0.0g, **Cholesterol** 20mg, **Sodium** 85mg, **Potassium** 150mg, **Total Carbohydrates** 1g, Fiber 0g, Sugar 0g, **Protein** 8g, **Phosphorus** 90mg

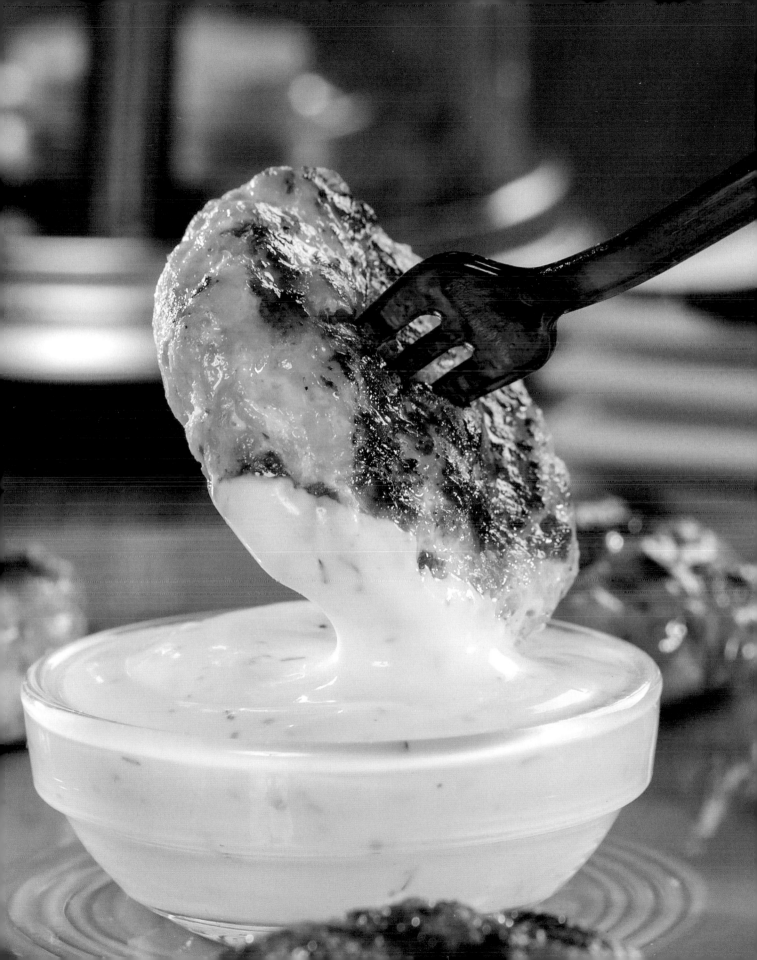

Deviled Eggs Italiano

Serves 12, 1 egg half per serving

6	hard-boiled eggs, peeled and cut in half lengthwise
1/3	cup light mayonnaise
2	tablespoons finely chopped sun-dried tomatoes, divided
1	tablespoon chopped fresh basil
1/2	teaspoon garlic powder

1 Separate egg whites and yolks. In a small bowl, finely mash egg yolks, then add mayonnaise, 1 tablespoon sun-dried tomatoes, basil, and garlic powder; mix well.

2 Evenly fill egg white halves with yolk mixture and place on a platter. Sprinkle remaining tomato pieces over the top of each egg. Cover with plastic wrap and refrigerate until ready to serve.

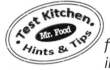

We found the easiest way to stuff deviled eggs is to place the filling in a resealable plastic bag, snip the corner, and pipe the filling into each egg white. That's how we do it here in the Test Kitchen.

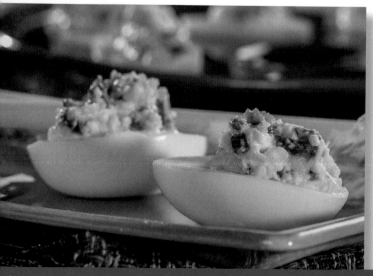

Choices/Exchanges, 1/2 carbohydrate, 1 lean protein

Calories 70, Calories From Fat 30, **Total Fat** 3.5g, Saturated Fat 1.0g, Trans Fat 0.0g, **Cholesterol** 120mg, **Sodium** 230mg, **Potassium** 360mg, **Total Carbohydrates** 6g, Fiber 1g, Sugar 4g, **Protein** 5g, **Phosphorus** 80mg

Baked Parmesan Zucchini Chips

Serves 6, about 4 chips per serving

1/2	cup whole-wheat seasoned bread crumbs
1	tablespoon shredded Parmesan cheese
1/2	teaspoon garlic powder
1/4	teaspoon salt
1/4	teaspoon black pepper
2	zucchini
1	tablespoon reduced-fat mayonnaise

1 Preheat oven to 425°F. Lightly coat a baking sheet with cooking spray.

2 In a small bowl, mix bread crumbs, cheese, garlic powder, salt, and pepper; set aside.

3 Cut zucchini into 1/2-inch slices and place in a single layer on prepared baking sheet. Spread a thin layer of mayonnaise on each zucchini slice. Top with bread crumb mixture.

4 Bake 15 to 20 minutes, or until browned on top. Serve immediately.

Did You Know?
Whole-wheat bread crumbs have 20% less carbs than traditional bread crumbs, plus they have more than double the fiber.

Choices/Exchanges, 1/2 starch, 1 nonstarchy vegetable

Calories 60, Calories From Fat 15, **Total Fat** 1.5g, Saturated Fat 0.0g, Trans Fat 0.0g, **Cholesterol** 0mg, **Sodium** 330mg, **Potassium** 180mg, **Total Carbohydrates** 9g, Fiber 2g, Sugar 2g, **Protein** 3g, **Phosphorus** 35mg

10-Minute Tuscan Bruschetta

Serves 8, 1 slice per serving

1	cup seeded and chopped Roma tomatoes
1/4	teaspoon salt
2	tablespoons balsamic vinegar
8	(1/2-inch thick) diagonal slices French bread
2	cloves garlic
2	tablespoons slivered fresh basil
4	tablespoons olive oil

1 Preheat broiler. Line a baking sheet with foil.

2 In a small bowl, mix tomatoes, salt, and balsamic vinegar; set aside.

3 Place bread on prepared baking sheet and toast until lightly browned. Rub each slice with garlic clove.

4 Spoon tomatoes evenly over bread, top with basil, and drizzle with olive oil. Serve immediately.

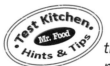

Test Kitchen, Mr. Food, Hints & Tips

If you love garlic, then you'll love this tip. When you rub a clove of peeled garlic over toasted bread, the coarse texture of the bread acts like a fine grater and leaves just a hint of garlic evenly over the surface. That means lots of taste and no extra calories or fat.

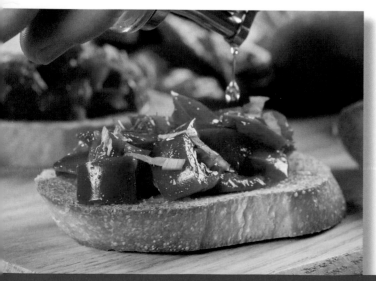

Choices/Exchanges, 2 starch, 1 1/2 fat

Calories 240, Calories From Fat 80, **Total Fat** 9.0g, Saturated Fat 1.5g, Trans Fat 0.0g, **Cholesterol** 0mg, **Sodium** 460mg, **Potassium** 135mg, **Total Carbohydrates** 35g, Fiber 2g, Sugar <1g, **Protein** 6g, **Phosphorus** 75mg

Crunchy Munchy Green Beans

Serves 10, 3 green beans per serving

30	fresh green beans, trimmed
1/4	cup all-purpose flour
2	eggs
2	tablespoons low-fat milk
1	cup bread crumbs
1/2	teaspoon onion powder
1/4	teaspoon garlic powder
1/8	teaspoon cayenne pepper
1/8	teaspoon salt
	Cooking spray

1 In a large saucepan, cover beans with water. Bring to a boil, and boil 5 minutes or until crisp-tender; drain. Plunge beans into ice water to stop them from cooking; drain again and pat dry.

2 Place flour in a shallow dish. In a shallow bowl, whisk eggs and milk. In another shallow bowl, mix bread crumbs, onion powder, garlic powder, cayenne pepper, and salt.

3 Preheat oven to 425°F. Coat a baking sheet with cooking spray.

4 Toss green beans in flour, shaking off excess. One at a time, dip them in egg mixture, then dredge in bread-crumb mixture. Place on prepared baking sheet, then coat beans with cooking spray.

5 Bake 15 minutes or until golden.

Just a Thought

Could these be the perfect snack? They're baked, not fried. They have the crunch and taste we crave. And, if that isn't enough, they have less than 0.5 g of saturated fat and less than 12 g of carbs per serving. Yes, these are quite possibly the perfect snack!

Choices/Exchanges, 1 carbohydrate

Calories 80, Calories From Fat 20, **Total Fat** 2.0g, Saturated Fat 0.0g, Trans Fat 0.0g, **Cholesterol** 40mg, **Sodium** 125mg, **Potassium** 80mg, **Total Carbohydrates** 12g, Fiber 1g, Sugar 1g, **Protein** 3g, **Phosphorus** 50mg

Cheesy Garlic & Herb Stuffed Tomatoes

Serves 6, 4 tomato halves per serving

12	grape or cherry tomatoes, cut in half lengthwise, with seeds and flesh removed
4	ounces fat-free cream cheese, softened
1/4	teaspoon minced garlic
2	teaspoons chopped fresh chives

1 Place tomato halves on a serving platter.

2 In a bowl, mix the remaining ingredients until well combined. Spoon evenly into tomato halves. Refrigerate until ready to serve.

Test Kitchen Hints & Tips — Mr. Food

A shortcut to remove the seeds and flesh of the tomatoes is to use a melon baller. Now for an easy way to fill the tomatoes, place cream cheese mixture in a resealable plastic bag, snip off the corner, and squeeze the mixture into each tomato just as we did to fill our Deviled Eggs Italiano (see page 24).

Choices/Exchanges, 1 nonstarchy vegetable

Calories 25, Calories From Fat 0, **Total Fat** 0.0g, Saturated Fat 0.0g, Trans Fat 0.0g, **Cholesterol** 0mg, **Sodium** 105mg, **Potassium** 110mg, **Total Carbohydrates** 3g, Fiber 0g, Sugar 0g, **Protein** 3g, **Phosphorus** 80mg

Mama Mia Meatballs

Serves 12, 2 meatballs per serving

1	pound lean hot Italian turkey sausage, casings removed
1/2	cup plain dry bread crumbs
1/3	cup grated Parmesan cheese
1/4	cup water
1/4	cup coarsely chopped fresh parsley
1	egg
1-1/4	teaspoons garlic powder
1/2	teaspoon black pepper

1 Preheat oven to 350°F. Coat a rimmed baking sheet with cooking spray.

2 In a large bowl, combine all ingredients; mix well. Form mixture into 24 (1-inch) meatballs and place on prepared baking sheet.

3 Bake 25 to 30 minutes, or until no pink remains, turning the meatballs over halfway through baking.

Serving Suggestion

Just like peanut butter and jelly is the perfect combo, we think our meatballs are best when teamed with some warmed low-sodium marinara sauce for dipping. Mama mia, now that's good eating!

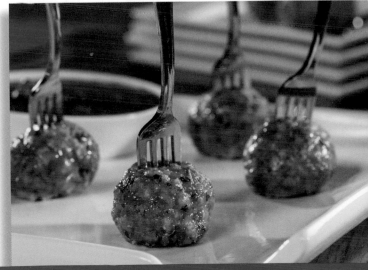

Choices/Exchanges, 1 lean protein, 1 fat

Calories 90, Calories From Fat 45, **Total Fat** 5.0g, Saturated Fat 1.5g, Trans Fat 0.0g, **Cholesterol** 20mg, **Sodium** 380mg, **Potassium** 30mg, **Total Carbohydrates** 4g, Fiber 0g, Sugar 0g, **Protein** 8g, **Phosphorus** 40mg

Crab-Stuffed Mushrooms

Serves 4, 3 mushrooms per serving

12	large mushrooms (about 3/4 pound), cleaned (see Tip)
1	tablespoon olive oil
1/2	small onion, finely chopped
1/2	medium red bell pepper, finely chopped
1	(6.5-ounce) can lump crabmeat, drained and squeezed
1/4	cup seasoned bread crumbs
1/2	teaspoon garlic powder
1/4	teaspoon black pepper
1	tablespoon grated Parmesan cheese

1 Preheat oven to 350°F. Remove mushroom stems from caps; finely chop stems.

2 In a large skillet over medium heat, heat oil. Add mushroom stems, onion, and bell pepper; sauté until tender, about 5 minutes. Remove from heat. Gently fold in crabmeat, bread crumbs, garlic powder, and black pepper. Do not overmix.

3 With a teaspoon, stuff each mushroom cap with crabmeat mixture, sprinkle with Parmesan cheese, and place on a rimmed baking sheet.

4 Bake 20 to 25 minutes, or until mushrooms are tender and heated through. Serve immediately.

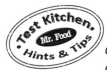

We found the best way to clean mushrooms is to wipe them with a damp towel. Mushrooms are very absorbent, so washing them can waterlog them and change their texture.

Choices/Exchanges, 1/2 starch, 1 nonstarchy vegetable, 1 lean protein, 1/2 fat

Calories 130, Calories From Fat 45, **Total Fat** 5.0g, Saturated Fat 1.0g, Trans Fat 0.0g, **Cholesterol** 40mg, **Sodium** 370mg, **Potassium** 470mg, **Total Carbohydrates** 10g, Fiber 2g, Sugar 2g, **Protein** 13g, **Phosphorus** 205mg

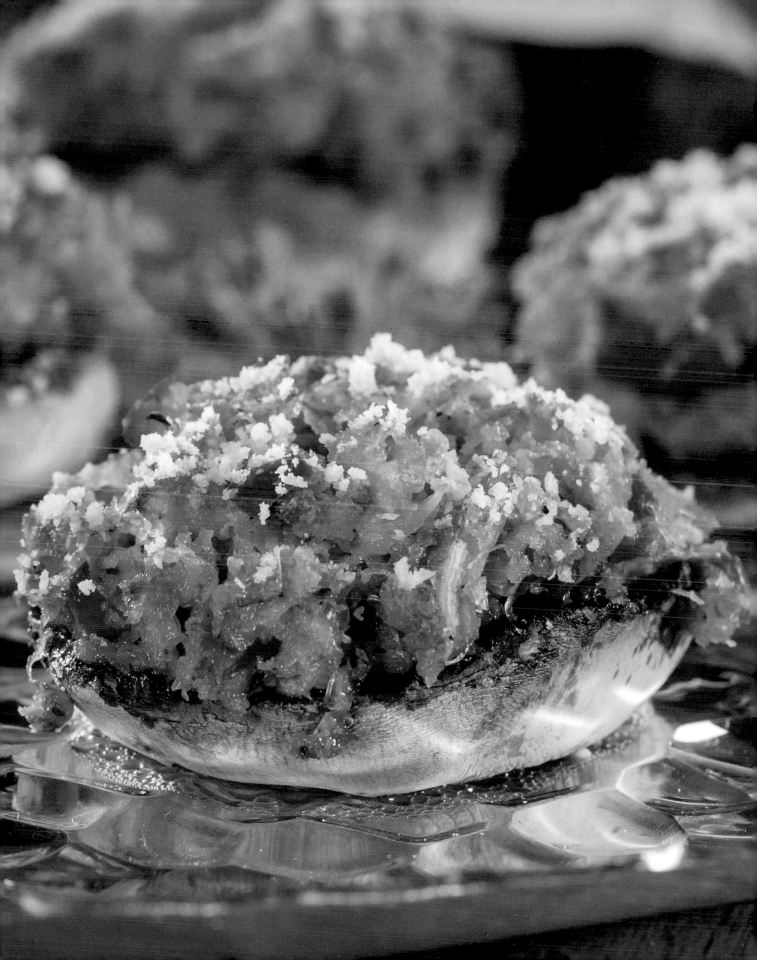

Bite-Sized Chicken & Waffles

Serves 12, 1 piece per serving

1/2   teaspoon garlic powder
1/4   teaspoon paprika
1/4   teaspoon salt
1/4   teaspoon black pepper
1/2   pound boneless, skinless chicken breasts, cut into 1/2-inch slices
1/4   cup sugar-free pancake syrup
1   tablespoon butter, melted
3   frozen whole-wheat waffles

1 In a small bowl, combine garlic powder, paprika, salt, and pepper; mix well. Sprinkle chicken evenly with seasoning mixture.

2 In another small bowl, mix syrup and melted butter; set aside.

3 In a skillet coated with cooking spray, over high heat, cook chicken 5 to 6 minutes, or until no pink remains.

4 Meanwhile, toast waffles. Cut each waffle into quarters and place on a serving platter. Place a slice of chicken on top of each waffle piece and drizzle with the syrup mixture. Serve immediately.

Good for You!
Chicken and waffles is a Southern favorite that is as down-home as can be. Our lightened-up version cuts down on over 3/4 of the fat, calories, and carbs.

Choices/Exchanges, 1/2 starch, 1 lean protein

Calories 70, Calories From Fat 20, **Total Fat** 2.0g, Saturated Fat 1.0g, Trans Fat 0.0g, **Cholesterol** 15mg, **Sodium** 180mg, **Potassium** 65mg, **Total Carbohydrates** 8g, Fiber <1g, Sugar 1g, **Protein** 6g, **Phosphorus** 50mg

Party Shrimp Egg Rolls

Serves 12, 2 egg rolls per serving

1/4	cup lower-sodium soy sauce
2	tablespoons light brown sugar
1	teaspoon ground ginger
1	teaspoon garlic powder
3	cups finely shredded Napa cabbage (see Tip)
1	small carrot, peeled and shredded
2	scallions, chopped
4	ounces frozen salad shrimp, thawed, drained, and coarsely chopped
24	wonton wrappers (not egg roll wrappers)
1	egg, lightly beaten
	Cooking spray

1 In a small bowl, combine soy sauce, brown sugar, ginger, and garlic powder; mix well.

2 In a large bowl, combine cabbage, carrot, scallions, and shrimp; mix well. Pour soy sauce mixture over cabbage mixture, toss to coat well, and let stand 10 minutes. Place cabbage mixture in a colander and squeeze to drain well.

3 Preheat oven to 450°F. Coat a baking sheet with cooking spray.

4 Spoon about 1 tablespoon cabbage mixture evenly onto center of each wrapper. Lightly brush edges with beaten egg. Fold one corner of each wrapper up over cabbage mixture, then fold both sides over, envelope style; roll up tightly. Place on prepared baking sheet. Spray a light coating of cooking spray over rolls.

5 Bake 12 to 15 minutes, or until crispy. Serve immediately.

Test Kitchen. Mr. Food Hints & Tips

Not sure what Napa cabbage is? Well, it's also referred to as Chinese cabbage and is found in most produce departments. But just in case you don't see it, you can always use finely shredded green cabbage. The key here is to make sure it is finely shredded.

Choices/Exchanges, 1 carbohydrate

Calories 80, Calories From Fat 10, **Total Fat** 1.0g, Saturated Fat 0.0g, Trans Fat 0.0g, **Cholesterol** 35mg, **Sodium** 135mg, **Potassium** 90mg, **Total Carbohydrates** 14g, Fiber <1g, Sugar 3g, **Protein** 4g, **Phosphorus** 45mg

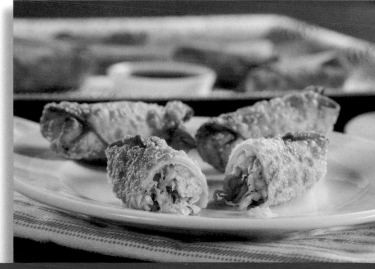

Chesapeake-Style Shrimp

Serves 8, about 3 shrimp per serving

1-1/2	tablespoons butter, melted
1	teaspoon seafood seasoning
4	garlic cloves, minced
1/4	cup chopped fresh parsley
1	pound large shrimp (24 to 30 count), peeled and deveined

1 Preheat oven to 350°F. Coat a 9 × 13-inch baking dish with cooking spray.

2 In a large bowl, mix butter, seafood seasoning, and garlic. Add parsley and shrimp; toss to coat. Spread in a single layer in prepared baking dish.

3 Bake 15 to 20 minutes, or until shrimp turn pink, turning halfway through cooking. Serve immediately.

Did You Know?
If you're wondering about the numbers after the shrimp in the list of ingredients, it's the size of the shrimp we think works best. It means there are 24 to 30 shrimp per pound. The lower the count, the larger the shrimp.

Choices/Exchanges, 2 lean protein

Calories 80, Calories From Fat 25, **Total Fat** 3.0g, Saturated Fat 1.5g, Trans Fat 0.0g, **Cholesterol** 90mg, **Sodium** 105mg, **Potassium** 120mg, **Total Carbohydrates** 1g, Fiber 0g, Sugar 0g, **Protein** 12g, **Phosphorus** 120mg

Chicken & Broccoli Quiche Bites

Serves 12, 2 quiche bites per serving

1	cup (4 ounces) fat-free shredded Cheddar cheese
3/4	cup frozen chopped broccoli, thawed and well drained
1/2	cup diced cooked chicken breast
1/4	cup chopped onion
2/3	cups fat-free milk
2	eggs
1/3	cup pancake & baking mix
1/4	teaspoon salt
1/8	teaspoon black pepper

1 Preheat oven to 400°F. Coat two (12-cup) mini-muffin tins with cooking spray.

2 In a large bowl, mix cheese, broccoli, chicken, and onion. Divide mixture evenly into muffin cups.

3 In another bowl, beat milk, eggs, baking mix, salt, and pepper until smooth. Pour evenly into muffin cups.

4 Bake 15 to 20 minutes, or until set. Let stand 5 minutes before removing from muffin tins.

Did You Know?

These can be made a day or two before you plan on serving them and simply reheated when needed. Now that's the kind of shortcut we all need when hosting a get-together.

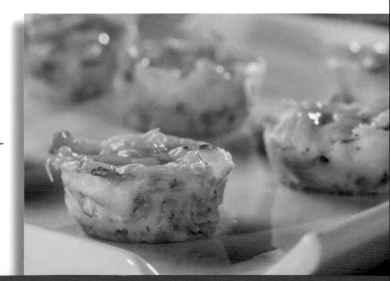

Choices/Exchanges, 1 lean protein, 1/2 fat

Calories 80, Calories From Fat 30, **Total Fat** 3.5g, Saturated Fat 1.5g, Trans Fat 0.0g, **Cholesterol** 45mg, **Sodium** 180mg, **Potassium** 80mg, **Total Carbohydrates** 4g, Fiber 0g, Sugar <1g, **Protein** 6g, **Phosphorus** 70mg

Your Very Own Tortilla Chips

Serves 8, about 14 chips per serving

1	tablespoon canola oil
3	tablespoons lime juice
1	(12-ounce) package corn tortillas
1	teaspoon onion powder
1	teaspoon ground cumin
1	teaspoon chili powder
1	teaspoon salt
1/4	teaspoon black pepper

1 Preheat oven to 350°F. Lightly coat 2 to 3 baking sheets with cooking spray.

2 In a small bowl, combine oil and lime juice. Lightly brush on both sides of each tortilla.

3 Cut each tortilla into 8 wedges and arrange in a single layer on prepared baking sheets.

4 In a small bowl, combine onion powder, cumin, chili powder, salt, and pepper. Sprinkle evenly over chips.

5 Bake 7 minutes. Rotate pans and bake 7 to 8 more minutes, or until chips are crisp but not too brown. Serve immediately, or let cool and store in an airtight container.

Serving Suggestion

Sure you can serve these naked (them, not you!), but try teaming them up with our Cowboy Hummus (see page 42) or Guacamole with a Twist (see page 41).

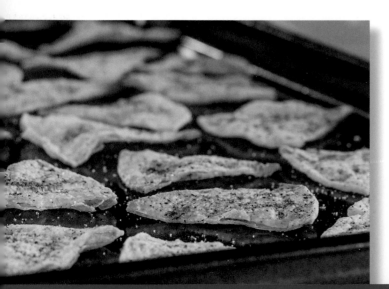

Choices/Exchanges, 1 1/2 starch

Calories 110, Calories From Fat 25, **Total Fat** 3.0g, Saturated Fat 0.0g, Trans Fat 0.0g, **Cholesterol** 0mg, **Sodium** 300mg, **Potassium** 85mg, **Total Carbohydrates** 21g, Fiber 2g, Sugar 0g, **Protein** 3g, **Phosphorus** 135mg

Beefed-Up Empanadas

Serves 10, 2 empanadas per serving

1/2	pound 95% extra-lean ground beef
1/4	cup finely chopped onion
1/2	teaspoon cumin
1/2	teaspoon garlic powder
1/4	teaspoon salt
1/4	teaspoon black pepper
1/4	cup frozen corn, thawed
1/3	cup salsa
2	tablespoons tomato sauce
20	wonton wrappers
	Cooking spray

1 Preheat oven to 400°F. Coat baking sheet(s) with cooking spray.

2 In a large, nonstick skillet, cook ground beef, onion, cumin, garlic powder, salt, and pepper 5 to 7 minutes, or until beef is browned; drain. Add corn, salsa, and tomato sauce, and cook until heated through. Set aside to cool.

3 Working with 1 wonton wrapper at a time, spoon 1 teaspoon beef mixture into center of each wrapper. Using your finger, wet the edge of wrapper with water. Fold wrapper over diagonally, forming a triangle. Using a fork, press to seal edges of wrapper. Place on prepared baking sheet(s) and repeat with remaining wrappers and filling. Coat lightly with cooking spray.

4 Bake 5 to 6 minutes per side, or until golden, turning once.

Serving Suggestion

Serve these like they do south of the border by putting out bowls of fresh salsa and sour cream (reduced fat, of course) for dipping. This is practically the beginning of a fiesta. Olé!

Choices/Exchanges, 1 starch

Calories 90, Calories From Fat 15, **Total Fat** 1.5g, Saturated Fat 0.5g, Trans Fat 0.0g, **Cholesterol** 15mg, **Sodium** 200mg, **Potassium** 135mg, **Total Carbohydrates** 11g, Fiber <1g, Sugar <1g, **Protein** 7g, **Phosphorus** 65mg

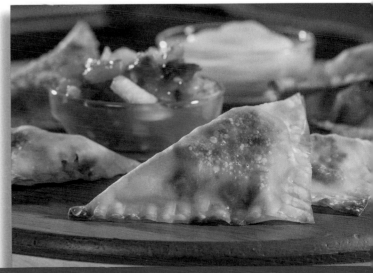

Athenian Pizza

Serves 12, 1 slice per serving

1	tablespoon olive oil
1	onion, thinly sliced
1	(10-ounce) package prebaked whole-wheat pizza crust
4	ounces roasted red peppers, patted dry and sliced
3	tablespoons sliced black olives
1/2	cup crumbled reduced-fat feta cheese
1	teaspoon Italian seasoning

1 In a large skillet over medium heat, heat oil. Add onion and cook 15 to 20 minutes, or until golden and caramelized, stirring frequently.

2 Preheat oven to 400°F.

3 Place pizza crust on round pizza pan. Top with onion, roasted peppers, olives, and feta cheese. Sprinkle with Italian seasoning

4 Bake 8 to 10 minutes, or until crust is crisp. Cut into 12 slices and serve immediately.

Test Kitchen. Mr. Food Hints & Tips

Caramelizing onions brings out their natural sugars and makes them taste unbelievably good. So ya won't wanna skip this step. And since the feta and olives add a touch of saltiness, there's no need for any added salt.

Choices/Exchanges, 1 starch, 1/2 fat

Calories 90, Calories From Fat 35, **Total Fat** 4.0g, Saturated Fat 1.5g, Trans Fat 0.0g, **Cholesterol** <5mg, **Sodium** 200mg, **Potassium** 30mg, **Total Carbohydrates** 13g, Fiber 2g, Sugar 1g, **Protein** 4g, **Phosphorus** 5mg

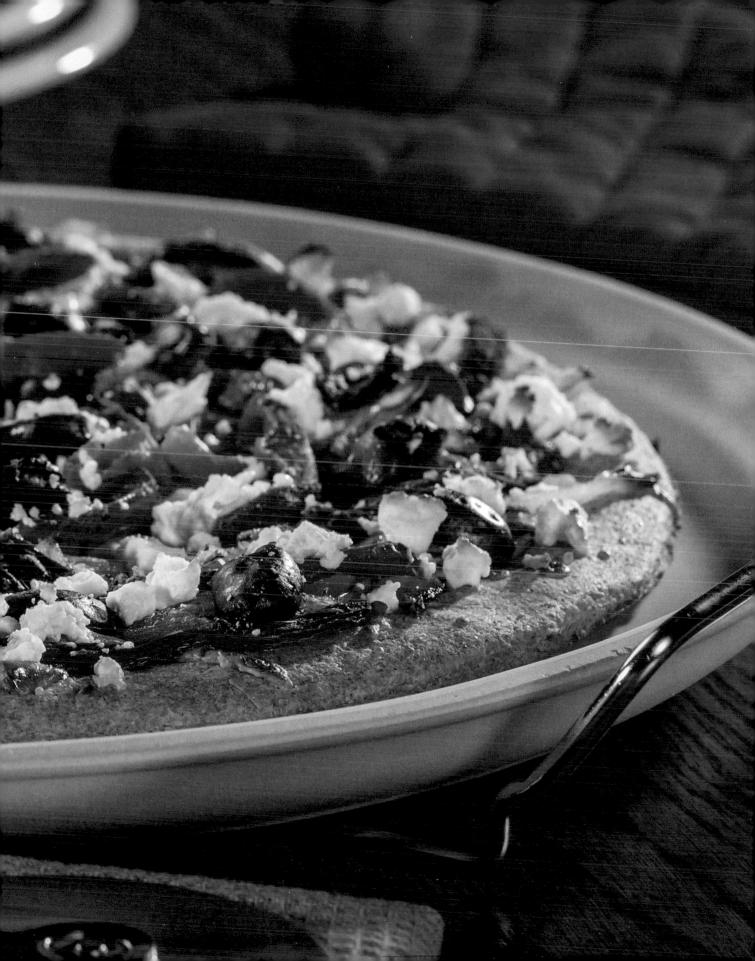

Everyone's Favorite Party Dip

Serves 20, 1-1/2 tablespoons per serving

1	(14-ounce) can artichoke hearts in water, drained, squeezed dry, and chopped
1/2	(12-ounce) jar roasted red peppers, patted dry and chopped
1/3	cup trans-fat-free mayonnaise
3	ounces reduced-fat cream cheese, softened
1	cup shredded reduced-fat pepper-jack cheese, divided

1 Preheat oven to 350°F. Coat a 9-inch pie plate with cooking spray.

2 In a bowl, combine all ingredients, except 1/2 cup pepper-jack cheese. Spoon into prepared pie plate. Sprinkle with remaining cheese.

3 Bake 15 to 20 minutes, or until mixture is bubbly and heated through.

Serving Suggestion

Instead of serving this with the normal salty crackers or chips, try serving it with gluten-free crackers and/or lots of fresh-cut veggies. That will certainly help you stay on track!

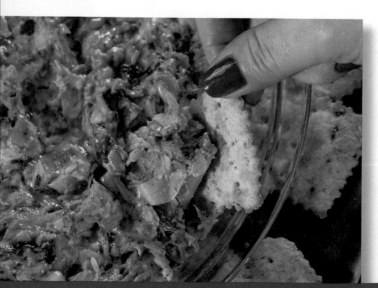

Choices/Exchanges, 1/2 fat

Calories 30, Calories From Fat 10, **Total Fat** 1.0g, Saturated Fat 0.0g, Trans Fat 0.0g, **Cholesterol** <5mg, **Sodium** 90mg, **Potassium** 95mg, **Total Carbohydrates** 3g, Fiber 1g, Sugar 0g, **Protein** 3g, **Phosphorus** 45mg

Guacamole with a Twist

Serves 8, about 1/4 cup per serving

24	medium spears fresh asparagus, trimmed and roughly chopped
4	ounces reduced-fat cream cheese
1/2	cup salsa
2	teaspoons lime juice
2	tablespoons chopped fresh cilantro
2	cloves garlic
1/4	cup chopped red onion
1/4	teaspoon salt

1 Place asparagus in a pot with enough water to cover. Bring to a boil and cook 5 minutes, or until very tender. Drain and rinse with cold water.

2 In a food processor or blender, place asparagus and the remaining ingredients; process until smooth. Refrigerate 1 hour, or until chilled.

Just a Thought
We often try to create recipes with unexpected ingredients, and we'd say using asparagus in this guacamole recipe is definitely unexpected (and delicious).

Choices/Exchanges, 1/2 carbohydrate, 1/2 fat

Calories 50, Calories From Fat 25, **Total Fat** 2.5g, Saturated Fat 1.5g, Trans Fat 0.0g, **Cholesterol** 10mg, **Sodium** 190mg, **Potassium** 170mg, **Total Carbohydrates** 5g, Fiber 1g, Sugar 2g, **Protein** 3g, **Phosphorus** 50mg

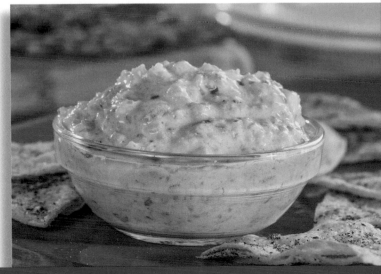

Cowboy Hummus

Serves 12, 2-1/2 tablespoons per serving

2	(15-ounce) cans kidney beans, drained, with 1/4 cup liquid reserved
1	tomato, cut into chunks and seeds removed
3	garlic cloves
2	tablespoons olive oil
1	teaspoon cumin
1	teaspoon chili powder
1/4	teaspoon salt
1/2	cup fresh cilantro

1 Combine all ingredients in a food processor. Process until mixture is smooth and creamy and no lumps remain, scraping down sides of bowl as needed.

2 Serve immediately, or cover and refrigerate until ready to serve.

Good for You!
Did you know that kidney beans are packed with lots of good-for-you fiber and protein, plus they help regulate our body's glucose level for hours after eating them?

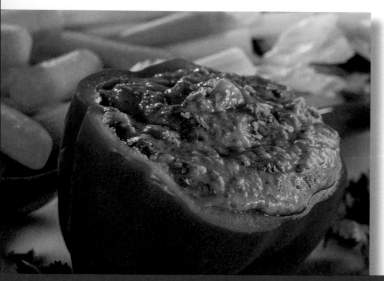

Choices/Exchanges, 1 carbohydrate, 1/2 fat

Calories 90, Calories From Fat 25, **Total Fat** 2.5g, Saturated Fat 0.0g, Trans Fat 0.0g, **Cholesterol** 0mg, **Sodium** 290mg, **Potassium** 230mg, **Total Carbohydrates** 12g, Fiber 5g, Sugar 0g, **Protein** 4g, **Phosphorus** 75mg

Sensational Salads

Confetti Quinoa Toss

Serves 6, about 3/4 cup per serving

1-1/2	cups water
1	cup uncooked quinoa, rinsed
1/4	cup finely chopped red onion
1/4	cup chopped yellow bell pepper
1/4	cup chopped red bell pepper
1/4	cup chopped fresh cilantro
3	tablespoons lime juice
1/2	cup finely diced carrots
1/4	cup slivered almonds
1/2	cup chopped dried apricots
1/2	jalapeño pepper, seeded and finely diced
1/8	teaspoon salt
1/8	teaspoon black pepper

1 In a saucepan over medium-high heat, bring water to a boil. Add quinoa, reduce heat to low, cover, and simmer 15 to 20 minutes, or until water is absorbed. Transfer to a serving bowl and refrigerate until cold.

2 Once quinoa is cold, add the remaining ingredients and toss. Refrigerate at least 1 hour before serving. Fluff with a fork when ready to serve.

Good for You!
Quinoa is a great source of protein, plus it's cholesterol-free and low fat. One cup has more than 8 grams of protein and only 245 calories. Now that's something to smile about!

Choices/Exchanges, 1 1/2 starch, 1/2 fruit, 1 fat

Calories 190, Calories From Fat 40, **Total Fat** 4.5g, Saturated Fat 0.5g, Trans Fat 0.0g, **Cholesterol** 0mg, **Sodium** 65mg, **Potassium** 440mg, **Total Carbohydrates** 32g, Fiber 5g, Sugar 10g, **Protein** 6g, **Phosphorus** 185mg

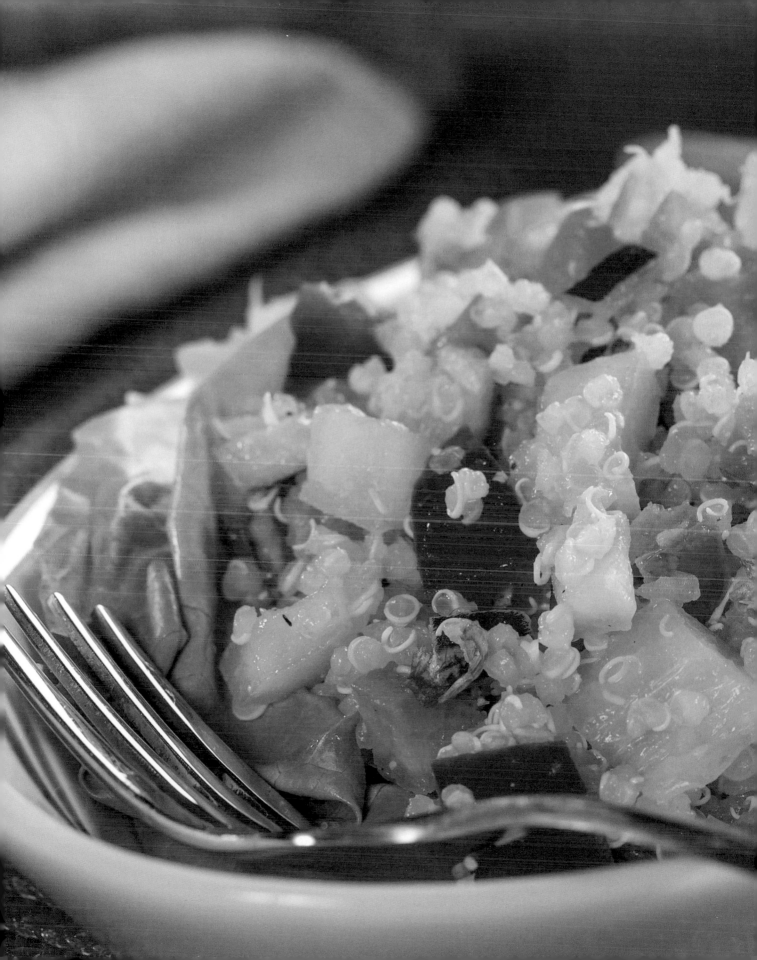

Greek Vegetable Salad

Serves 8, about 1/2 cup per serving

Dressing

1/4	cup olive oil
1/4	cup red wine vinegar
1	clove garlic, minced
1	tablespoon sugar
2	teaspoons dried oregano
1/2	teaspoon dry mustard
1/4	teaspoon salt
1/4	teaspoon black pepper

Salad

1	pound asparagus, trimmed and cut into bite-sized pieces
1	red bell pepper, diced
1	(14-ounce) can artichoke hearts, drained and roughly chopped
1-1/2	cups grape tomatoes
2	ounces reduced-fat feta cheese crumbles

1 In a jar with a tight-fitting lid, combine all dressing ingredients and shake well; set aside.

2 In a large skillet over high heat, bring about 3 cups water to a simmer. Add asparagus and cook 60 to 90 seconds, or just until crisp-tender. Drain and rinse with cold water to stop the cooking. Once cool and well drained, transfer to a large bowl.

3 Stir in bell pepper, artichoke hearts, and tomatoes.

4 Pour half the dressing over the salad and stir to coat. Add in feta cheese and toss gently. Toss with remaining dressing. Cover salad and refrigerate at least 30 minutes before serving.

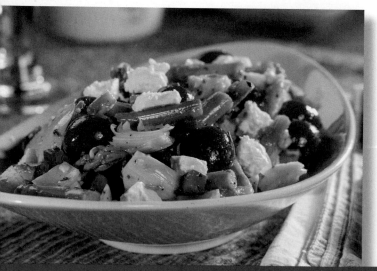

Test Kitchen, Mr. Food Hints & Tips

If you would like, you can add some pitted Greek olives to this for a blast of flavor. Of course, it's up to you.

Choices/Exchanges, 2 vegetable, 2 fat

Calories 130, Calories From Fat 80, **Total Fat** 9.0g, Saturated Fat 2.0g, Trans Fat 0.0g, **Cholesterol** 5mg, **Sodium** 210mg, **Potassium** 410mg, **Total Carbohydrates** 13g, Fiber 5g, Sugar 3g, **Protein** 5g, **Phosphorus** 35mg

Harvest Kale Salad

Serves 6, about 1 cup per serving

6	cups fresh kale, chopped into bite-sized pieces
3	tablespoons olive oil
3	tablespoons lemon juice
1/2	teaspoon salt
1/4	teaspoon black pepper
2	tablespoons reduced-fat grated Parmesan cheese
3	tablespoons chopped pecans
1/3	cup dried cranberries

1 Place kale in a large bowl. Drizzle olive oil and lemon juice over leaves. Using your hands, squeeze the kale and massage the dressing into the leaves. This will soften the leaves and is very important.

2 Sprinkle with salt, pepper, and Parmesan cheese, and toss to combine. Add pecans and cranberries and toss gently. Serve immediately, or keep refrigerated until ready to serve.

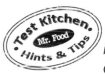 *Test Kitchen. Mr. Food Hints & Tips*

This is one salad that not only holds up well once the dressing is added, we actually think it tastes better if you do make it ahead of time.

Choices/Exchanges, 1/2 fruit, 1 vegetable, 2 fat

Calories 150, Calories From Fat 100, **Total Fat** 11.0g, Saturated Fat 1.5g, Trans Fat 0.0g, **Cholesterol** 0mg, **Sodium** 260mg, **Potassium** 360mg, **Total Carbohydrates** 13g, Fiber 2g, Sugar 10g, **Protein** 4g, **Phosphorus** 90mg

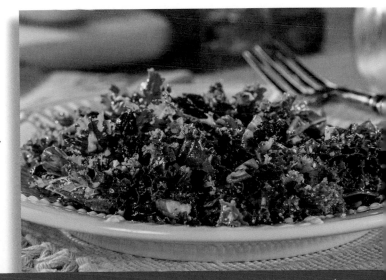

Cashew-Studded Grapefruit Salad

Serves 6, about 1-1/2 cups per serving

1	(6-ounce) bag chopped romaine lettuce
1	large grapefruit, peeled and cut into sections
1/2	red onion, thinly sliced
1/4	cup light balsamic vinaigrette
3	tablespoons chopped cashews

1 In a large bowl, combine lettuce, grapefruit sections, and onion.

2 Toss with dressing and sprinkle with cashews. Serve immediately.

Test Kitchen. Mr. Food Hints & Tips

The easiest way to peel a grapefruit is to cut off about 1/4 inch from the top and bottom. Then sit the grapefruit on one of the cut ends (this way it won't roll around). Now cut the skin off starting at the top in a downward motion. Turn and cut until all the skin is removed, and voilà, a perfectly peeled grapefruit, the white part (pith) and all.

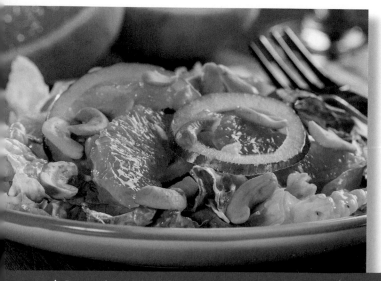

Choices/Exchanges, 1/2 fruit, 1 vegetable, 1/2 fat

Calories 70, Calories From Fat 30, **Total Fat** 3.5g, Saturated Fat 0.5g, Trans Fat 0.0g, **Cholesterol** 0mg, **Sodium** 120mg, **Potassium** 220mg, **Total Carbohydrates** 9g, Fiber 2g, Sugar 4g, **Protein** 2g, **Phosphorus** 40mg

Grilled Bistro Salad

Serves 4, about 2 cups per serving

1/2	pound boneless, skinless chicken breasts
1/2	pound fresh asparagus, trimmed
1	(5-ounce) package mixed baby greens
1-1/2	cups grape tomatoes, halved
1/4	cup frozen corn, thawed
1/4	cup crumbled feta cheese
1/4	cup sliced almonds, toasted
1/4	cup chopped dates
1/4	cup low-fat raspberry vinaigrette

1 Preheat grill to medium.

2 Place chicken and asparagus on grill. Grill chicken 5 to 6 minutes per side, or until no longer pink, and grill asparagus until tender.

3 Remove from grill; set aside asparagus and cut chicken into bite-sized pieces.

4 In a large bowl, toss together the remaining ingredients. Top with chicken and asparagus, drizzle with dressing, and serve.

Test Kitchen. Mr. Food Hints & Tips

Look for dates in the produce section of your local grocery store. (We're talking about the dried fruit, not someone to share your salad with.) If you can't find them there, they're often next to the raisins and dried cranberries.

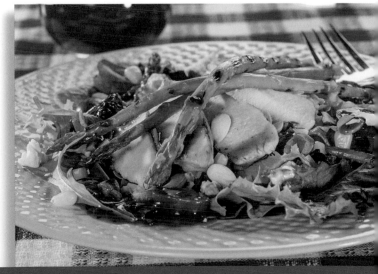

Choices/Exchanges, 1/2 fruit, 1 vegetable, 2 lean protein, 1 1/2 fat

Calories 210, Calories From Fat 80, **Total Fat** 9.0g, Saturated Fat 2.0g, Trans Fat 0.0g, **Cholesterol** 40mg, **Sodium** 230mg, **Potassium** 480mg, **Total Carbohydrates** 16g, Fiber 3g, Sugar 10g, **Protein** 18g, **Phosphorus** 215mg

Our Favorite BLT Salad

Serves 6, about 2 cups per serving

3/4	cup fat-free mayonnaise
3/4	cup buttermilk
1	tablespoon minced onion
1	tablespoon chopped fresh parsley
1/2	teaspoon garlic powder
1/8	teaspoon black pepper
1	large head romaine lettuce, cut into bite-sized pieces
2	large tomatoes, chopped
1/2	pound reduced-sodium turkey bacon, cooked and coarsely chopped
1	cup seasoned whole-wheat croutons

1 In a medium bowl, combine mayonnaise, buttermilk, onion, parsley, garlic powder, and pepper. Refrigerate at least 1 hour.

2 Meanwhile, in a large bowl, combine lettuce, tomatoes, bacon, and croutons. Toss with dressing and serve immediately.

Good for You!

With a name like buttermilk and its creamy texture, most people assume that it's loaded with butter and fat. Surprise! That is far from the truth. Actually it is extremely low in fat and calories and is a great choice when you are trying to eat healthy.

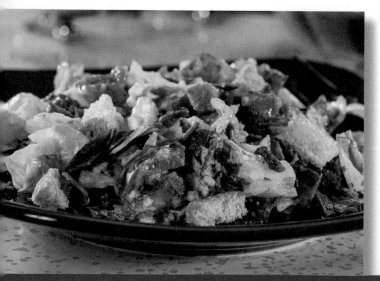

Choices/Exchanges, 1/2 starch, 1 vegetable, 1 medium-fat protein, 1/2 fat

Calories 160, Calories From Fat 50, **Total Fat** 6.0g, Saturated Fat 2.0g, Trans Fat 0.0g, **Cholesterol** 30mg, **Sodium** 540mg, **Phosphorus** 100mg, **Total Carbohydrates** 17g, Fiber 5g, Sugar 7g, **Protein** 9g, **Potassium** 570mg

Company Fancy Stacked Salad

Serves 8, about 2-1/2 cups per serving

1	head romaine lettuce, cut into bite-sized pieces
3	tomatoes, chopped and seeded
1	orange or yellow bell pepper, cut into bite-sized pieces
3	celery stalks, chopped
6	radishes, chopped
1	(10-ounce) package frozen green peas, thawed
4	hard-boiled eggs, peeled and chopped
1	cup (4 ounces) fat-free shredded Cheddar cheese
1	cup reduced-fat ranch dressing

1 In a large glass salad or trifle bowl, layer all ingredients in the order of the ingredients list except the dressing. Serve immediately, or cover and refrigerate until ready to serve. Right before serving, drizzle with dressing and dig in.

Just a Thought
This is a great salad for when you're having company over since it's so darn colorful. The best part is that it's not only diabetes friendly, it tastes even better than it looks.

Choices/Exchanges, 1/2 starch, 1 vegetable, 1 lean protein, 1 fat

Calories 160, Calories From Fat 50, **Total Fat** 6.0g, Saturated Fat 1.0g, Trans Fat 0.0g, **Cholesterol** 125mg, **Sodium** 360mg, **Potassium** 600mg, **Total Carbohydrates** 16g, Fiber 5g, Sugar 6g, **Protein** 12g, **Phosphorus** 155mg

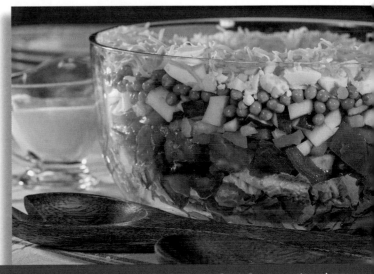

Farmer's Chow Chow Relish

Serves 10, about 1 cup per serving

2 cups frozen cauliflower, thawed and cut into small pieces
2 cups frozen sliced carrots, thawed
2 cups frozen cut green beans, thawed
1 (15-ounce) can red kidney beans, rinsed and drained
1 large onion, coarsely chopped
1/2 red bell pepper, cut into 1/2-inch pieces
2 cups water
1 cup white vinegar
1/2 cup sugar
1/2 cup granulated Splenda
1/2 teaspoon celery seed
1/4 teaspoon turmeric
1/2 teaspoon salt

1 In a large, heat-proof bowl, combine cauliflower, carrots, green beans, kidney beans, onion, and bell pepper; set aside.

2 In a medium saucepan over high heat, bring the remaining ingredients to a boil, stirring occasionally. Pour over vegetables; mix gently to coat.

3 Let mixture sit until cool; stir again, and then cover and refrigerate until ready to serve.

Test Kitchen, Mr. Food Hints & Tips

We saved a lot of time making this by starting with frozen vegetables. Not only are they often fresher than fresh veggies, using the frozen ones saves us from having to prep and blanch fresh ones.

Choices/Exchanges, 1/2 starch, 1/2 carbohydrate, 2 vegetable

Calories 110, Calories From Fat 0, **Total Fat** 0.0g, Saturated Fat 0.0g, Trans Fat 0.0g, **Cholesterol** 0mg, **Sodium** 290mg, **Potassium** 330mg, **Total Carbohydrates** 25g, Fiber 5g, Sugar 13g, **Protein** 4g, **Phosphorus** 70mg

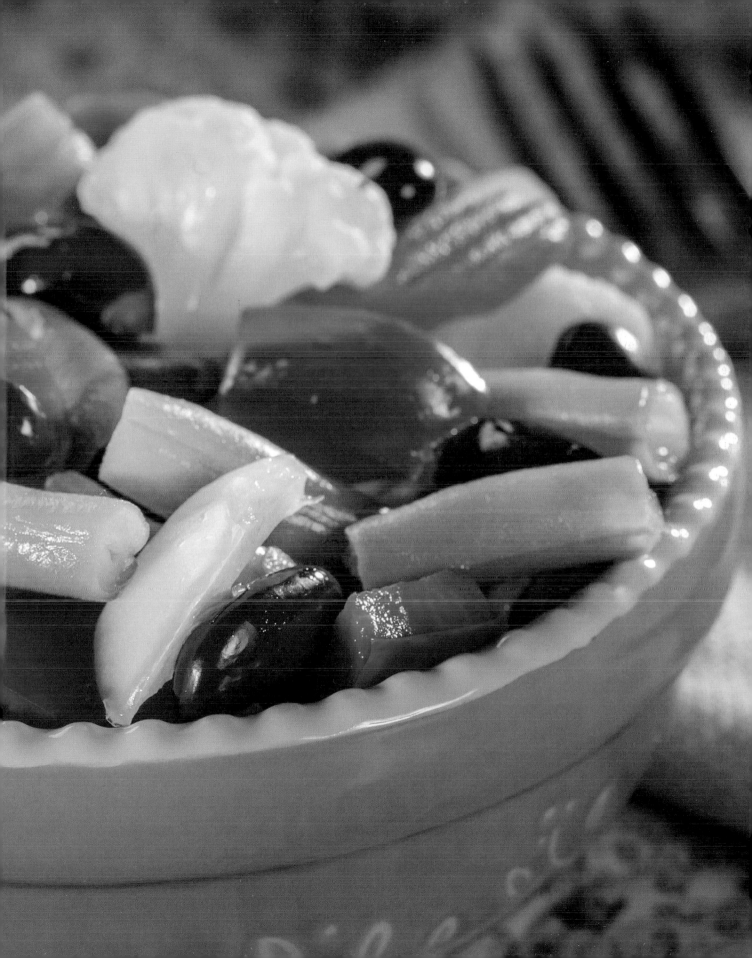

Johnny Apple Slaw

Serves 8, about 3/4 cup per serving

1/2	large apple, cored and diced
1	teaspoon lemon juice
1	(16-ounce) bag shredded coleslaw mix (tri-color, if available)
1	celery stalk, diced
1/2	cup finely chopped onion
2-1/2	cups frozen corn, thawed
1/4	cup olive oil
1/4	cup apple cider vinegar
2	tablespoons sugar
3/4	teaspoon salt

1 Sprinkle cut apple with lemon juice to prevent browning. In a large bowl, toss together the coleslaw mix, apple, celery, onion, and corn.

2 In a small bowl, combine the remaining ingredients; pour over coleslaw mixture and toss well.

3 Cover and refrigerate 1 hour, or until ready to serve. Toss again before serving.

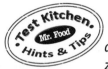

Although you can use almost any apple in this recipe, we think a tart apple like the Granny Smith adds just the right amount of zing. Let us know what you think on Facebook, please!

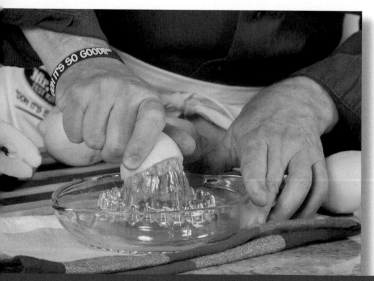

Choices/Exchanges, 1/2 starch, 1/2 carbohydrate, 1 vegetable, 1 fat

Calories 140, Calories From Fat 60, **Total Fat** 7.0g, Saturated Fat 1.0g, Trans Fat 0.0g, **Cholesterol** 0mg, **Sodium** 240mg, **Potassium** 290mg, **Total Carbohydrates** 19g, Fiber 3g, Sugar 7g, **Protein** 2g, **Phosphorus** 50mg

Caprese Pasta Salad

Serves 4, about 1 cup per serving

2	cups cooked small shell-shaped pasta, rinsed and drained
1-1/2	cups cherry or grape tomatoes, halved
3	reduced-fat mozzarella string cheese sticks, cut into 1/2-inch pieces
2	tablespoons slivered fresh basil
1/2	cup reduced-fat balsamic vinaigrette

1 In a large bowl, combine pasta, tomatoes, cheese, and basil. Toss with dressing.

2 Cover and refrigerate 1 hour, or until ready to serve. Toss again before serving.

Did You Know?
The colors of the tomatoes, basil, and mozzarella represent the red, green, and white of the Italian flag. Saluting not required!

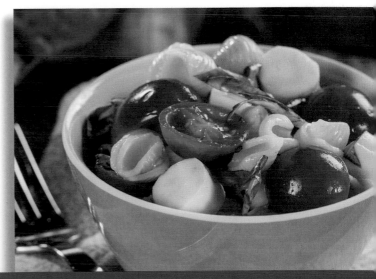

Choices/Exchanges, 1 1/2 starch, 1 vegetable, 1 fat

Calories 180, Calories From Fat 50, **Total Fat** 6.0g, Saturated Fat 1.0g, Trans Fat 0.0g, **Cholesterol** <5mg, **Sodium** 400mg, **Potassium** 180mg, **Total Carbohydrates** 26g, Fiber 1g, Sugar 1g, **Protein** 6g, **Phosphorus** 0mg

Cucumber Dill Chill

Serves 6, about 3/4 cup per serving

1/2	cup rice vinegar
1/2	teaspoon salt
2	teaspoons granulated Splenda
1/4	cup water
2-1/4	cups thinly sliced cucumbers
1/2	onion, thinly sliced
1/2	red bell pepper, slivered
1	tablespoon fresh dill

1 In a bowl, combine vinegar, salt, Splenda, and water. Add cucumbers, onion, red bell pepper, and dill. Toss gently to combine.

2 Cover and refrigerate 1 hour, or until ready to serve. Toss again before serving.

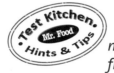

You can thinly slice the cucumbers with a sharp knife, a mandoline, or a food processor. Either way you'll love how fresh tasting this is.

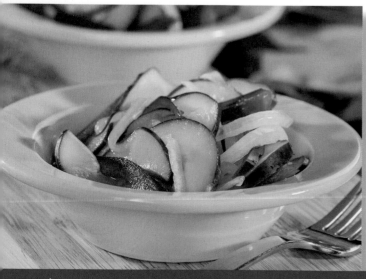

Choices/Exchanges, 1 vegetable

Calories 20, Calories From Fat 0, **Total Fat** 0.0g, Saturated Fat 0.0g, Trans Fat 0.0g, **Cholesterol** 0mg, **Sodium** 200mg, **Potassium** 120mg, **Total Carbohydrates** 4g, Fiber 1g, Sugar 3g, **Protein** 1g, **Phosphorus** 20mg

Kickin' Shrimp & Avocado Salad

Serves 4, about 1/2 cup per serving

2	tablespoons lime juice
1	teaspoon olive oil
1/8	teaspoon salt
1/8	teaspoon black pepper
2	avocados
1	cup frozen cooked salad shrimp, thawed
1	tomato, diced
1/4	cup chopped red onion
1	tablespoon finely diced jalapeño pepper
1	tablespoon chopped cilantro

1 In a small bowl, combine lime juice, oil, salt, and pepper; set aside.

2 Cut avocados in half, remove pits, and carefully scoop avocado meat out of skins; set aside skins for serving. Cut avocado flesh into cubes and place in a large bowl. Add shrimp, tomato, onion, jalapeño, and cilantro, then gently toss with lime juice mixture.

3 Refrigerate at least 15 minutes before serving. When ready to serve, spoon salad into reserved avocado skins.

Did You Know?
If you like hot stuff, look for jalapeños with some white lines on their skin. That usually means they're more mature and tend to be hotter.

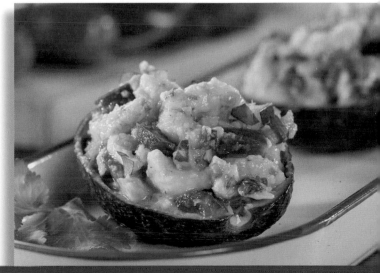

Choices/Exchanges, 1/2 carbohydrate, 1 lean protein, 2 1/2 fat

Calories 190, Calories From Fat 130, **Total Fat** 14.0g, Saturated Fat 2.0g, Trans Fat 0.0g, **Cholesterol** 70mg, **Sodium** 250mg, **Potassium** 590mg, **Total Carbohydrates** 10g, Fiber 6g, Sugar 2g, **Protein** 10g, **Phosphorus** 190mg

Mediterranean Couscous

Serves 12, about 1/4 cup per serving

1	(10-ounce) package Moroccan couscous (see note)
1	(15-ounce) can chickpeas, drained and rinsed
1	teaspoon dried oregano
1/2	cup chopped red onion
2	tomatoes, chopped
1/4	cup sliced black olives
1/2	cup lemon juice
2	tablespoons olive oil
1	teaspoon salt
1/2	teaspoon black pepper
2	tablespoons chopped fresh parsley

1 Prepare couscous according to package directions. Place in a serving bowl and let cool.

2 Once cool, add the remaining ingredients; toss until well combined.

3 Cover and refrigerate at least 1 hour, or until ready to serve. Fluff with a fork before serving.

Did You Know?
Here we've used Moroccan couscous, but we've also tried using Israeli couscous with equally tasty results. You just have to adjust cooking time, as Israeli couscous is larger and takes longer to cook.

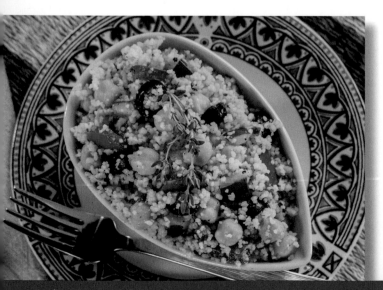

Choices/Exchanges, 2 starch, 1/2 fat

Calories 160, Calories From Fat 25, **Total Fat** 3.0g, Saturated Fat 0.0g, Trans Fat 0.0g, **Cholesterol** 0mg, **Sodium** 330mg, **Potassium** 180mg, **Total Carbohydrates** 29g, Fiber 3g, Sugar 1g, **Protein** 5g, **Phosphorus** 80mg

Thai Broccoli Salad

Serves 4, about 1-3/4 cups per serving

3	tablespoons creamy, natural unsweetened peanut butter
2	teaspoons sesame oil
1	tablespoon white vinegar
1	tablespoon lower-sodium soy sauce
1	teaspoon sugar
1/4	teaspoon ground ginger
1/8	teaspoon salt
6	cups broccoli florets, steamed
1	red bell pepper, cut into thin strips
1/2	cup thinly sliced red onion
1/8	teaspoon red pepper flakes

1 In a small bowl, whisk together peanut butter and sesame oil. Add vinegar, soy sauce, sugar, ginger, and salt; set aside.

2 In a large bowl, combine broccoli, bell pepper, and onion. Pour dressing over vegetables and toss until well coated. Sprinkle with red pepper flakes and toss to combine.

3 Cover and refrigerate 1 hour, or until ready to serve. Toss before serving.

Good for You!
Not familiar with natural unsweetened peanut butter? You can find it either with the other peanut butters or in the organic aisle of your favorite market.

Choices/Exchanges, 1/2 carbohydrate, 2 vegetable, 2 fat

Calories 130, Calories From Fat 60, **Total Fat** 7.0g, Saturated Fat 1.5g, Trans Fat 0.0g, **Cholesterol** 0mg, **Sodium** 180mg, **Potassium** 520mg, **Total Carbohydrates** 14g, Fiber 1g, Sugar 4g, **Protein** 7g, **Phosphorus** 125mg

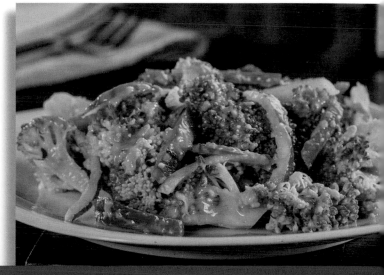

Guilt-Free Caesar Dressing

Serves 6, 1-1/2 tablespoons per serving

1/3	cup fat-free mayonnaise
2	tablespoons lemon juice
2	tablespoons fat-free milk
1	teaspoon Dijon-style mustard
2	tablespoons grated Parmesan cheese
1	clove garlic, minced
1/4	teaspoon black pepper

1 In a small bowl, stir together all ingredients. Chill until ready to use.

Good for You!

By using a few good-for-us substitutes, we cut the calories by more than 80% and the fat by more than 90% compared with traditional Caesar dressing. Now that's good news!

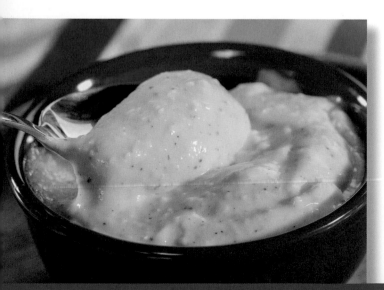

Choices/Exchanges, Free food

Calories 20, Calories From Fat 10, **Total Fat** 1.0g, Saturated Fat 0.0g, Trans Fat 0.0g, **Cholesterol** <5mg, **Sodium** 140mg, **Potassium** 30mg, **Total Carbohydrates** 3g, Fiber 0g, Sugar 1g, **Protein** <1g, **Phosphorus** 20mg

Easy Blender Green Goddess Dressing

Serves 12, 3 tablespoons per serving

1/2	cup white wine vinegar
1	bunch fresh parsley
6	scallions, sliced
2	cloves garlic
1	anchovy filet (optional)
3	tablespoons lemon juice
1	teaspoon salt (optional)
2	cups fat-free mayonnaise

1 In a blender, puree vinegar, parsley, scallions, garlic, anchovy, if desired, lemon juice, and salt, if desired, until well combined. Blend in mayonnaise.

2 Pour into a bowl. Cover and refrigerate 1 hour, or until ready to serve.

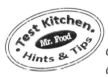

This makes a lot, but it will last up to a week in the fridge. You can use it on salad, to dip fresh veggies, or really, the possibilities are endless!

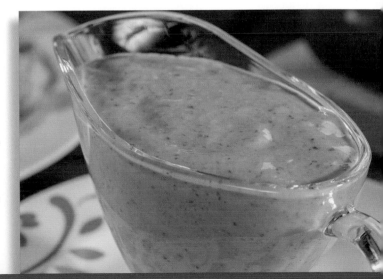

Choices/Exchanges, 1 carbohydrate

Calories 40, Calories From Fat 0, **Total Fat** 0.0g, Saturated Fat 0.0g, Trans Fat 0.0g, **Cholesterol** 0mg, **Sodium** 290mg, **Potassium** 140mg, **Total Carbohydrates** 11g, Fiber <1g, Sugar 0g, **Protein** <1g, **Phosphorus** 15mg

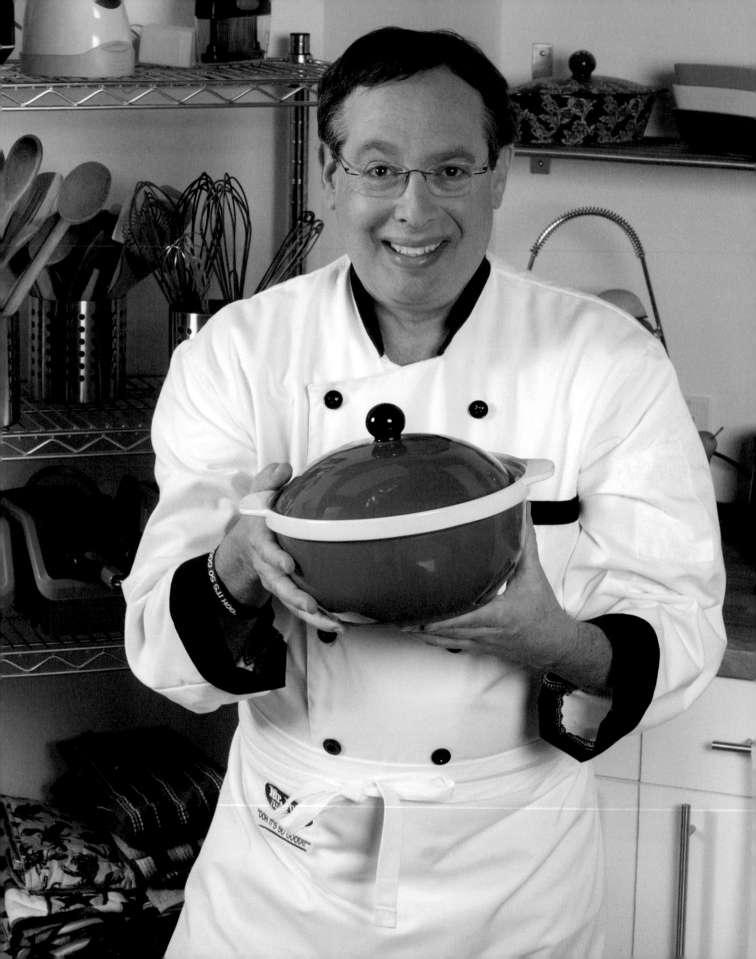

Warming Soups, Stews & Chilis

Down-Home Chicken & Dumplings

Serves 6, about 2/3 cup soup and 1 dumpling per serving

1/2	cup reduced-fat pancake & baking mix
3	tablespoons water
1/4	teaspoon dried rosemary, crushed
3-1/2	cups reduced-sodium chicken broth
1	tablespoon chopped fresh parsley
1-1/2	cups diced cooked chicken breast
1	cup frozen peas and carrots, thawed

1 In a medium bowl, stir together baking mix, water, and rosemary to make a soft dough.

2 In a soup pot over medium-high heat, bring broth and parsley to a boil.

3 Divide the dough into 6 equal pieces and drop into broth. Reduce heat to medium and cook, uncovered, 10 minutes.

4 Add chicken and vegetables; cover and simmer 10 more minutes, or until dumplings are thoroughly cooked.

Choices/Exchanges, 1 starch, 1 lean protein, 1/2 fat

Calories 140, Calories From Fat 35, **Total Fat** 4.0g, Saturated Fat 1.0g, Trans Fat 0.0g, **Cholesterol** 30mg, **Sodium** 220mg, **Potassium** 280mg, **Total Carbohydrates** 11g, Fiber 1g, Sugar 1g, **Protein** 15g, **Phosphorus** 200mg

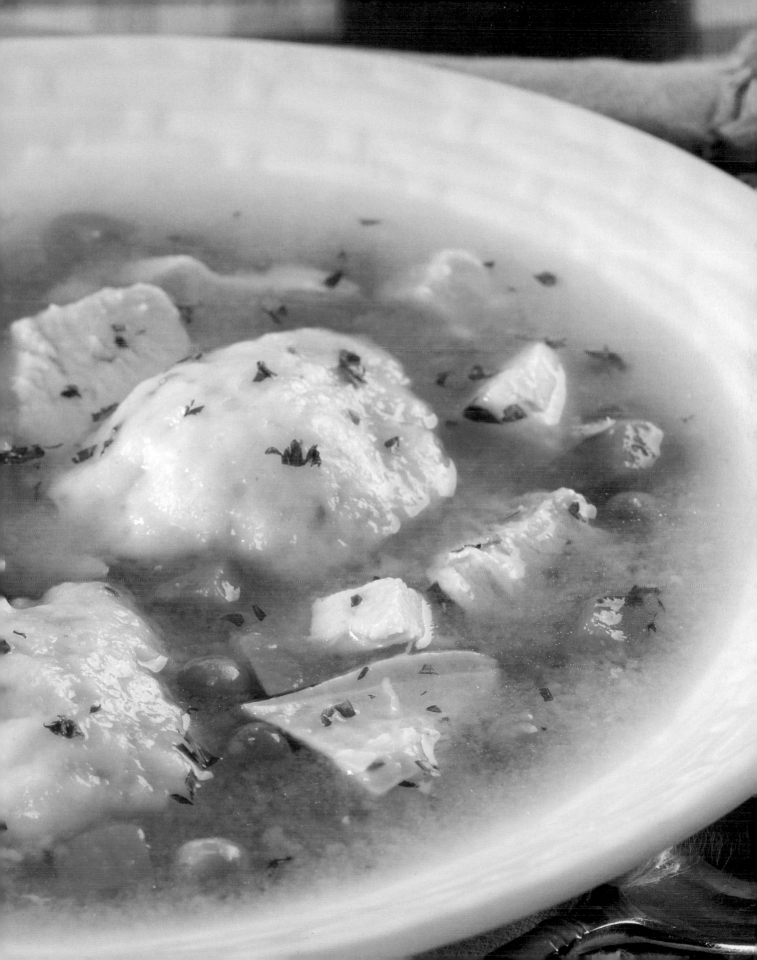

Aunt Nellie's Garden Soup

Serves 5, about 1-1/2 cups per serving

1	head cauliflower, cut into florets
5	carrots, peeled and cut into chunks
1	parsnip, peeled and cut into chunks
4	cups reduced-sodium chicken broth
4	cups water
1	teaspoon salt (optional)
1/4	teaspoon black pepper
1/4	teaspoon dried thyme
1	cup low-fat milk
2	tablespoons Parmesan cheese

1 In a soup pot, combine all ingredients except milk and Parmesan cheese. Bring to a boil over high heat. Reduce heat to low and simmer 30 minutes, or until vegetables are very tender.

2 Using an immersion blender (see Tip), puree until smooth. Stir in milk and simmer an additional 5 minutes, or until hot.

3 Spoon into bowls and top with Parmesan cheese.

Test Kitchen. Mr. Food Hints & Tips

An immersion blender is a huge time-saver all around the kitchen. If you don't have one, you could either pick one up (they are relatively inexpensive), or you can puree this in a food processor or blender, in batches. Pureeing is what makes this soup so smooth and silky without all the guilt.

Choices/Exchanges, 3 vegetable, 1/2 fat

Calories 110, Calories From Fat 15, **Total Fat** 1.5g, Saturated Fat 0.5g, Trans Fat 0.0g, **Cholesterol** <5mg, **Sodium** 530mg, **Potassium** 830mg, **Total Carbohydrates** 18g, Dietary Fiber 5g, Sugar 9g, **Protein** 7g, **Phosphorus** 165mg

Tuscan Minestrone

Serves 12, about 1-1/8 cups per serving

6	cups reduced-sodium beef broth
1	(28-ounce) can crushed tomatoes
1	(15.5-ounce) can Great Northern beans, undrained
1	(15.5-ounce) can red kidney beans, undrained
1	(9-ounce) package frozen mixed vegetables, thawed
1	(10-ounce) package frozen chopped spinach, thawed
1	small onion, chopped
1	teaspoon garlic powder
1	teaspoon Italian seasoning
1/2	teaspoon black pepper
1	cup uncooked ditalini or other small-shaped pasta

1 In a soup pot, combine all ingredients except the pasta. Bring to a boil over medium-high heat. Reduce heat to low and simmer 15 minutes.

2 Add pasta and simmer 10 more minutes, or until pasta is tender, stirring occasionally.

Serving Suggestion
Sprinkle with a bit of grated Parmesan cheese to add a special touch and a great pop of flavor.

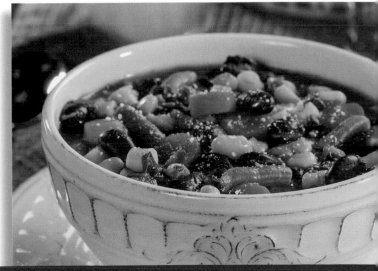

Choices/Exchanges, 1 starch, 3 nonstarchy vegetable

Calories 160, Calories From Fat 10, **Total Fat** 1.0g, Saturated Fat 0.0g, Trans Fat 0.0g, **Cholesterol** 0mg, **Sodium** 440mg, **Potassium** 570mg, **Total Carbohydrates** 30g, Fiber 7g, Sugar 1g, **Protein** 10g, **Phosphorus** 145mg

Rustic Peasant Soup

Serves 8, about 1 cup per serving

1	teaspoon olive oil
1	large onion, chopped
7	slices turkey bacon, cut into 1/2-inch pieces, cooked and drained
2	(15-ounce) cans chickpeas, rinsed
2	(14.5-ounce) cans no-salt-added diced tomatoes, undrained
4	cups reduced-sodium chicken broth
1/4	cup reduced-fat grated Parmesan cheese, divided
1	teaspoon garlic powder
1/4	teaspoon black pepper
6	cups loosely packed chopped kale

1 In a soup pot over medium-high heat, heat olive oil. Add onion and sauté about 5 minutes, or until translucent. Add bacon, chickpeas, tomatoes, broth, 2 tablespoons cheese, garlic powder, and pepper.

2 Reduce heat to medium-low and simmer about 20 minutes, stirring occasionally.

3 Add kale and simmer 10 more minutes. Sprinkle with remaining cheese and serve.

Good for You!

Kale is low in calories, high in fiber, and has zero fat. It's also packed with powerful antioxidants and is high in iron and vitamins A and K. It's definitely the perfect superfood for a diabetes-friendly diet.

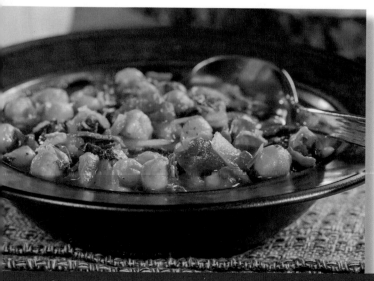

Choices/Exchanges, 1 starch, 4 vegetable, 1 fat

Calories 250, Calories From Fat 50, **Total Fat** 6.0g, Saturated Fat 1.5g, Trans Fat 0.0g, **Cholesterol** 10mg, **Sodium** 600mg, **Potassium** 800mg, **Total Carbohydrates** 38g, Fiber 7g, Sugar 4g, **Protein** 13g, **Phosphorus** 185mg

Heartied-Up Mac & Cheese Soup

Serves 6, about 1-1/8 cups per serving

2	teaspoons olive oil
3/4	cup chopped onion
1	teaspoon garlic powder
1	teaspoon dry mustard
1/2	teaspoon black pepper
4	cups reduced-sodium chicken broth
1	(16-ounce) package frozen broccoli cuts, thawed
1	tablespoon cornstarch
2/3	cup fat-free half-and-half
1/2	teaspoon salt (optional)
12	ounces cooked chicken breast, cut into bite-sized pieces
1	cup cooked elbow macaroni
3/4	cup reduced-fat shredded sharp Cheddar cheese

1 In a soup pot over medium heat, heat oil. Add onion and cook 3 to 4 minutes, or until soft. Add garlic powder, dry mustard, pepper, broth, and broccoli; bring to a boil. Reduce heat to low, cover, and simmer 8 to 10 minutes.

2 In a small bowl, whisk together the cornstarch and half-and-half. Add to soup, along with salt, if desired, chicken, and macaroni. Simmer 5 minutes, or until slightly thickened.

3 Stir in cheese. Cook 1 minute, or until cheese has melted, stirring constantly. Serve immediately.

Choices/Exchanges, 1/2 starch, 2 vegetable, 3 lean protein, 1/2 fat

Calories 250, Calories From Fat 70, **Total Fat** 8.0g, Saturated Fat 3.0g, Trans Fat 0.0g, **Cholesterol** 55mg, **Sodium** 550mg, **Potassium** 610mg, **Total Carbohydrates** 18g, Dietary Fiber 3g, Sugar 4g, **Protein** 27g, **Phosphorus** 345mg

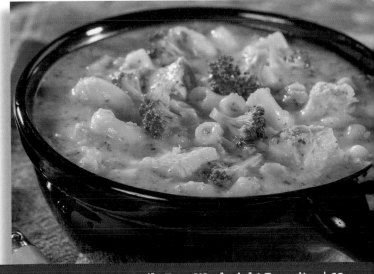

Skinny French Onion Soup

Serves 6, about 1 cup per serving

2	tablespoons olive oil
4	sweet onions, cut in half and thinly sliced
1/2	teaspoon dried thyme
1/4	cup red wine
1/3	cup apple cider
4	cups reduced-sodium beef broth
1/2	teaspoon salt (optional)
1/4	teaspoon black pepper
2	(1/2-inch thick) slices whole-grain bread
	Cooking spray
2	teaspoons grated Parmesan cheese

1 In a soup pot over medium heat, heat oil. Add onions and thyme and cook about 15 minutes, or until onions begin to brown.

2 Add red wine, apple cider, broth, salt, if desired, and pepper, and bring to a boil. Reduce heat to low and simmer 20 to 25 minutes.

3 Meanwhile, preheat oven to 350°F.

4 Place bread on a cutting board. Spray both sides with cooking spray, then cut into 1-inch pieces. Place in a small bowl and sprinkle with cheese; toss to coat evenly. Spread on a baking sheet and heat in oven, 5 to 7 minutes, or until bread is toasted. Serve immediately over the soup.

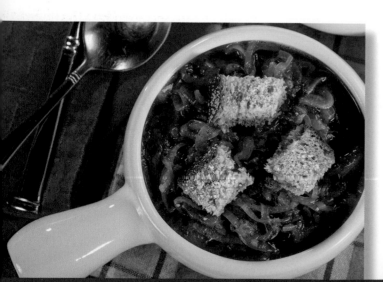

Test Kitchen. Mr. Food Hints & Tips

You want to take your time and make sure that your onions are really caramelized to a dark brown color. Caramelizing the onions brings out their natural sweetness and adds lots of flavor.

Choices/Exchanges, 1/2 carbohydrate, 1 vegetable, 1 fat

Calories 120, Calories From Fat 45, **Total Fat** 5.0g, Saturated Fat 1.0g, Trans Fat 0.0g, **Cholesterol** 0mg, **Sodium** 320mg, **Potassium** 150mg, **Total Carbohydrates** 15g, Fiber 2g, Sugar 5g, **Protein** 4g, **Phosphorus** 40mg

Veggie Bin Chowder

Serves 6, about 1 cup per serving

2	cups peeled, diced potatoes
1/2	cup chopped celery
1/2	cup diced carrots
1/2	cup chopped onion
3	cups reduced-sodium chicken broth
1-1/2	cups frozen corn
1	(12-ounce) can evaporated fat-free milk
3/4	cup reduced-fat shredded Cheddar cheese
1/2	teaspoon dried thyme
1/8	teaspoon black pepper
1	tablespoon cornstarch
2	tablespoons water
2	tablespoons bacon bits

1 In a soup pot over medium heat, combine potatoes, celery, carrots, onion, and broth. Bring to a boil, reduce heat to low, and cook 15 minutes, or until vegetables are tender. Stir in corn, evaporated milk, cheese, thyme, and pepper. Continue cooking 5 more minutes, or until the cheese has melted, stirring often.

2 In a small bowl, whisk together cornstarch and the water. Slowly stir into soup and cook 2 to 3 minutes, or until thickened. Stir in bacon bits and serve.

Test Kitchen Mr. Food Hints & Tips

We love this soup not only for its taste, but because it's a great way to clean out the veggie bin and turn all that goodness into a soup that's loaded with flavor and nutrients.

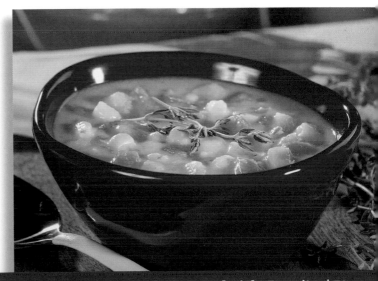

Choices/Exchanges, 1 starch, 1/2 fat-free milk, 1/2 fat

Calories 140, Calories From Fat 25, **Total Fat** 3.0g, Saturated Fat 1.5g, Trans Fat 0.0g, **Cholesterol** 10mg, **Sodium** 380mg, **Potassium** 530mg, **Total Carbohydrates** 19g, Fiber 1g, Sugar 9g, **Protein** 10g, **Phosphorus** 280mg

Irish Pub Potato Soup

Serves 4, about 1 cup per serving

2	cups reduced-sodium chicken broth
1	teaspoon minced garlic
1/2	cup chopped celery
1	cup shredded cabbage
2-1/2	cups fat-free milk
1	tablespoon light, trans-fat-free margarine
1-1/4	cups instant potato flakes
1/2	teaspoon onion powder
1/2	teaspoon salt
1/4	teaspoon black pepper
1/2	cup sliced scallions

1 In a soup pot over medium heat, combine broth, garlic, celery, and cabbage; bring to a boil. Reduce heat to low and cook about 10 minutes, or until vegetables are tender, stirring occasionally.

2 Add the remaining ingredients; mix well to combine. Cook 3 to 4 more minutes, or until soup thickens, stirring often.

Did You Know?
Adding potato flakes is a great way to thicken soups and sauces. Just don't overdo it. A little goes a long way.

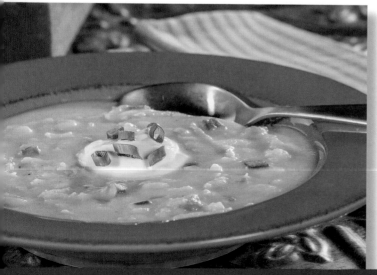

Choices/Exchanges, 1 starch, 1/2 fat-free milk, 1/2 fat

Calories 150, Calories From Fat 20, **Total Fat** 2.0g, Saturated Fat 0.5g, Trans Fat 0.0g, **Cholesterol** <5mg, **Sodium** 440mg, **Potassium** 660mg, **Total Carbohydrates** 24g, Fiber 2g, Sugar 10g, **Protein** 10g, **Phosphorus** 230mg

Protein-Packed Bean Soup

Serves 4, about 1 cup per serving

1	(15.5-ounce) can Great Northern beans, drained and rinsed
1	(15-ounce) can cannellini beans, undrained
2	cups low-sodium chicken broth
1/4	cup light, trans-fat-free margarine
2	large carrots, diced
1	(4-ounce) piece reduced-sodium deli ham, chopped
1/3	cup sliced scallions
1	bay leaf
1/4	teaspoon black pepper

1 In a soup pot, combine beans; mash slightly with a potato masher or back of a large spoon. Stir in broth and cook over low heat until heated through.

2 In a skillet over medium-high heat, melt margarine; sauté carrots until tender, stirring constantly. Add carrots, ham, scallions, bay leaf, and pepper to bean mixture. Cook over low heat 10 minutes, stirring occasionally. Discard bay leaf before serving.

Did You Know?

This soup has as much protein as a grilled chicken breast, 3 scrambled eggs, or a lean steak. Plus with no fat, beans might just be one of nature's healthiest foods.

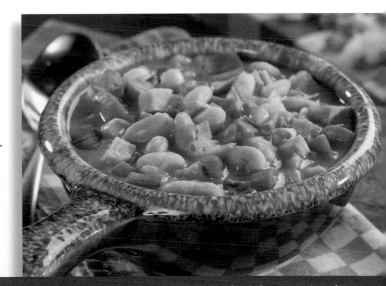

Choices/Exchanges, 2 starch, 1 vegetable, 2 lean protein

Calories 260, Calories From Fat 60, **Total Fat** 7.0g, Saturated Fat 1.5g, Trans 0.0g, **Cholesterol** 15mg, **Sodium** 540mg, **Potassium** 840mg, **Total Carbohydrates** 34g, Dietary Fiber 10g, Sugar 5g, **Protein** 18g, **Phosphorus** 285mg

Homestyle Lentil Soup

Serves 6, about 1 cup per serving

1	cup chopped carrots
1	cup chopped celery
1	cup finely chopped onion
1	cup dried lentils, rinsed and drained
4	cups reduced-sodium beef broth
3	cups water
1	teaspoon dried oregano
1	teaspoon garlic powder
1/2	teaspoon salt (optional)
1/2	teaspoon black pepper
2	cups fresh spinach, chopped

1. Coat a soup pot with cooking spray. Over medium heat, cook carrots, celery, and onion 6 to 8 minutes, or until tender, stirring occasionally.

2. Add lentils, broth, water, oregano, garlic powder, salt, if desired, and pepper. Mix well and bring to a boil over high heat. Reduce heat to low, cover, and simmer 50 to 60 minutes, or until lentils are tender, stirring occasionally.

3. Add spinach and cook 5 more minutes. Serve immediately.

Good for You!
Lentils are high in fiber, so not only has it been said that they lower cholesterol, but also that they prevent glucose levels from spiking after a meal. Oh, did we mention they taste great, too? Well they do!

Choices/Exchanges, 1 1/2 starch, 1 vegetable

Calories 150, Calories From Fat 0, **Total Fat** 0.0g, Saturated Fat 0.0g, Trans Fat 0.0g, **Cholesterol** 0mg, **Sodium** 310mg, **Potassium** 520mg, **Total Carbohydrates** 25g, Fiber 12g, Sugar 5g, **Protein** 12g, **Phosphorus** 170mg

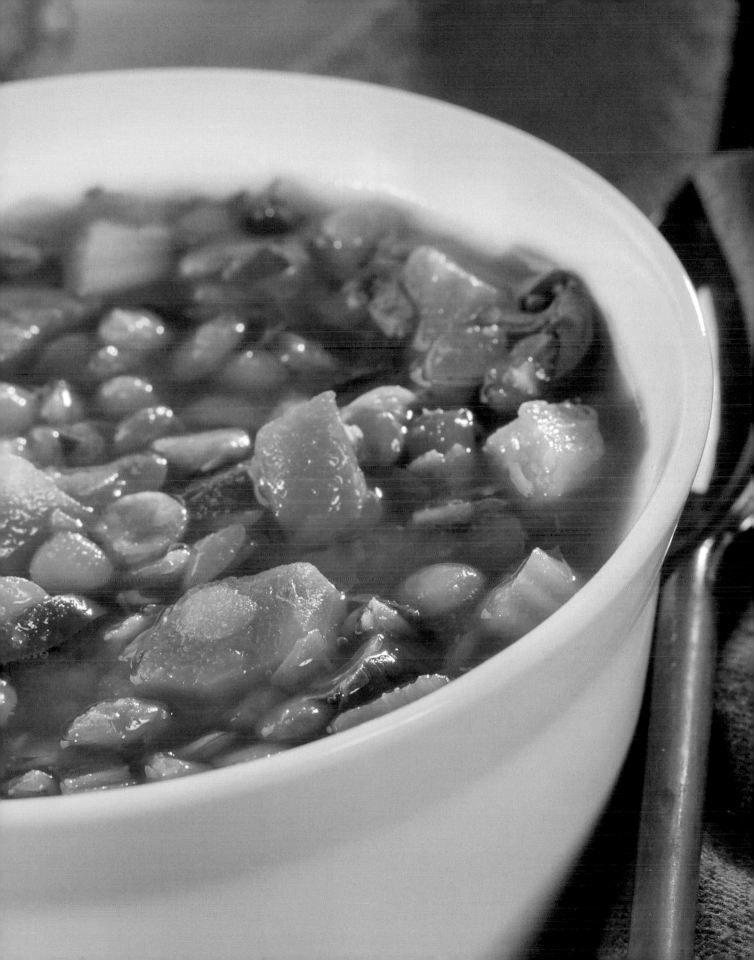

Sweet Potato & Ham Chowder

Serves 4, about 1-3/4 cups per serving

2 cups reduced-sodium chicken broth

1 sweet potato, peeled and diced

1 (14.5-ounce) can reduced-sodium diced tomatoes, undrained

1/2 cup chopped onion

1 (6-ounce) piece reduced-sodium deli ham, chopped

1 (12-ounce) can evaporated fat-free milk

3 tablespoons all-purpose flour

1 (8-ounce) can pineapple tidbits, in 100% pineapple juice, undrained

1 In a soup pot over high heat, bring broth, sweet potato, tomatoes, and onion to a boil. Cook 10 to 15 minutes, or until potato is tender.

2 Add ham, reduce heat to low, and simmer 5 minutes.

3 In a bowl, whisk together evaporated milk and flour until well combined. Add to soup mixture. Stir in pineapple and cook about 5 more minutes, or until soup has thickened and is heated through, stirring occasionally.

Did You Know?

The pineapple is the universal symbol of hospitality. That's why we can't think of a more welcoming way to bring your family to the table than with a bowl of this hearty fill-ya-up soup.

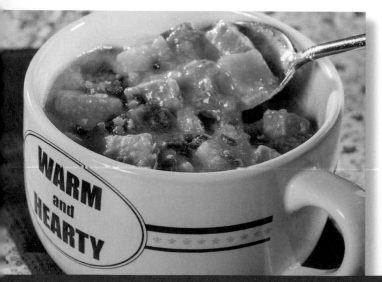

Choices/Exchanges, 1 fat-free milk, 1 1/2 carbohydrate, 1 lean protein

Calories 240, Calories From Fat 20, **Total Fat** 2.0g, Saturated Fat 0.0g, Trans Fat 0.0g, **Cholesterol** 20mg, **Sodium** 500mg, **Potassium** 830mg, **Total Carbohydrates** 38g, Fiber 3g, Sugar 24g, **Protein** 19g, **Phosphorus** 250mg

Creamy Tomato Rice Soup

Serves 4, about 1-1/2 cups per serving

2	(14.5-ounce) cans reduced-sodium diced tomatoes, undrained
1-3/4	cups reduced-sodium beef broth
1/4	cup water
1	cup fat-free dry milk powder
2	cups cooked brown rice
1	teaspoon dried basil
1/2	teaspoon salt (optional)
1/4	teaspoon black pepper

1 Place tomatoes with liquid in blender. Pulse 3 or 4 times, until still slightly chunky.

2 In a soup pot, combine broth and water, then slowly whisk in dry milk powder. Stir in tomatoes, rice, basil, salt, if desired, and pepper. Cook over medium-low heat 8 to 10 minutes, or until heated through. Serve immediately.

Good for You!
Did you know that brown rice has more than 4 times the fiber of white rice and is a great source of magnesium, which is good for our bones?

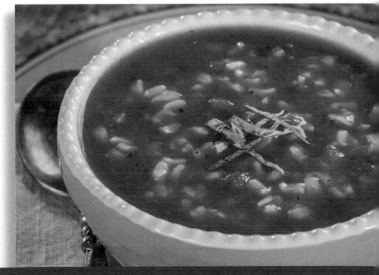

Choices/Exchanges, 1 1/2 starch, 1 fat-free milk, 2 vegetable

Calories 260, Calories From Fat 15, **Total Fat** 1.5g, Saturated Fat 0.0g, Trans Fat 0.0g, **Cholesterol** 5mg, **Sodium** 360mg, **Potassium** 1100mg, **Total Carbohydrates** 48g, Fiber 4g, Sugar 22g, **Protein** 16g, **Phosphorus** 405mg

Chicken & Wild Rice Soup

Serves 4, about 1-3/4 cups per serving

6	cups low-sodium chicken broth
1	cup chopped carrots
1	cup chopped celery
1/2	cup chopped onion
1	cup wild rice, rinsed
1/4	teaspoon poultry seasoning
1/8	teaspoon black pepper
1	cup diced cooked chicken breast

1 In a soup pot over high heat, combine broth, carrots, celery, and onion. Bring mixture to a boil, then stir in rice, poultry seasoning, and pepper.

2 Reduce heat to low, cover, and simmer 45 to 50 minutes, or until rice is tender, stirring occasionally.

3 Add chicken and cook about 5 more minutes, until soup is heated through.

Did You Know?
Wild rice isn't really rice. It's actually part of the grass family. However, it looks similar to rice, hence its name. There ya go, a bit of trivia to share with the family as you're all chowing down.

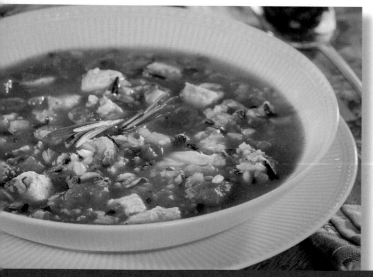

Choices/Exchanges, 2 starch, 2 vegetable, 2 lean protein

Calories 280, Calories From Fat 35, **Total Fat** 4.0g, Saturated Fat 1.0g, Trans Fat 0.0g, **Cholesterol** 30mg, **Sodium** 180mg, **Potassium** 780mg, **Total Carbohydrates** 40g, Fiber 4g, Sugar 4g, **Protein** 25g, **Phosphorus** 385mg

Strawberry Rhubarb Soup

Serves 4, about 3/4 cup per serving

4	cups frozen rhubarb, thawed
1-1/2	cups frozen strawberries, thawed
1/3	cup sugar
1/2	cup low-fat plain yogurt
1/8	teaspoon salt
1/4	cup chopped fresh mint

1 Place rhubarb, strawberries, sugar, yogurt, and salt in a blender; blend until smooth. Stir in mint and serve.

Did You Know?

No need to look for fresh rhubarb in the produce aisle because you should be able to find it in the freezer case next to the other frozen fruits. Actually, using frozen is a lot easier, and it's available year-round.

Choices/Exchanges, 2 carbohydrate

Calories 130, Calories From Fat 10, **Total Fat** 1.0g, Saturated Fat 0.0g, Trans Fat 0.0g, **Cholesterol** 0mg, **Sodium** 100mg, **Potassium** 530mg, **Total Carbohydrates** 29g, Fiber 4g, Sugar 23g, **Protein** 3g, **Phosphorus** 75g

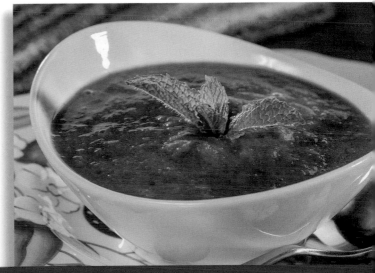

Chilled Watermelon Soup

Serves 5, about 1 cup per serving

6	cups cubed watermelon, divided
1/2	cup diced cucumber
6	tablespoons lime juice, divided
1	scallion, thinly sliced, divided
1/4	cup fat-free plain yogurt
1/2	jalapeño pepper, seeded and chopped
1/4	cup orange juice
1	teaspoon chopped fresh ginger
1/2	teaspoon salt

1 Dice 1 cup watermelon and combine in a bowl with cucumber, 2 tablespoons lime juice, and 1 tablespoon sliced scallion. Cover and refrigerate until ready to serve.

2 In a blender, place remaining watermelon, yogurt, remaining lime juice, remaining scallion, jalapeño, orange juice, ginger, and salt. Blend until smooth and creamy. Refrigerate about 2 hours, or until chilled.

3 Stir the reserved watermelon-cucumber mixture and divide evenly between five soup bowls.

4 Pour soup into bowls and serve.

Serving Suggestion
Want to fancy this up? Garnish each bowl with a dollop of yogurt and a bit of cilantro. It'll be picture-perfect.

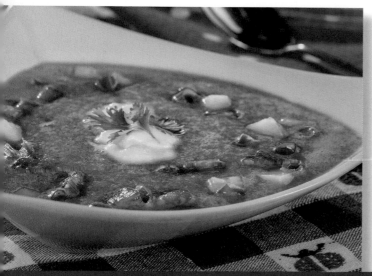

Choices/Exchanges, 1 carbohydrate

Calories 80, Calories From Fat 0, **Total Fat** 0.5g, Saturated Fat 0.0g, Trans Fat 0.0g, **Cholesterol** 0mg, **Sodium** 240mg, **Potassium** 340mg, **Total Carbohydrates** 19g, Fiber 1g, Sugar 13g, **Protein** 2g, **Phosphorus** 30mg

Burger & Tater Stew

Serves 8, about 1-1/8 cups per serving

1-1/2	pounds 95% extra-lean ground beef
1	onion, chopped
5	cups reduced-sodium beef broth
1	(14.5-ounce) can reduced-sodium diced tomatoes, undrained
2	russet baking potatoes, peeled and diced
2	cups frozen peas and carrots
1	teaspoon garlic powder
1/2	teaspoon black pepper
1	tablespoon cornstarch
2	tablespoons water

1 In a soup pot over medium-high heat, cook ground beef and onion 6 to 8 minutes, or until browned; drain excess liquid.

2 Add the remaining ingredients except cornstarch and water and bring to a boil. Reduce heat to medium and cook 15 to 20 minutes, or until potatoes are tender.

3 In a small bowl, whisk cornstarch and water. Stir into stew and simmer 5 more minutes, or until slightly thickened.

Serving Suggestion

This one is definitely for the meat and potato lovers in the crowd. Try topping off each bowl with a little drizzle of ketchup or mustard. They're fat-free and full of flavor.

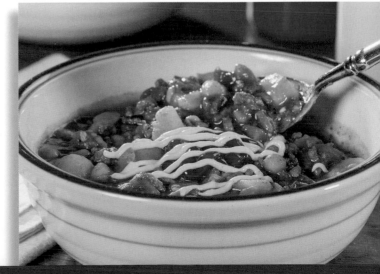

Choices/Exchanges, 1 starch, 3 lean protein

Calories 200, Calories From Fat 40, **Total Fat** 4.5g, Saturated Fat 2.0g, Trans Fat 0.0g, **Cholesterol** 55mg, **Sodium** 340mg, **Potassium** 720mg, **Total Carbohydrates** 17g, Fiber 3g, Sugar 3g, **Protein** 23g, **Phosphorus** 225mg

Farmhouse Beef Stew

Serves 6, about 1-1/2 cups per serving

2	tablespoons all-purpose flour
1	pound well-trimmed beef stew meat, cut into 1-inch chunks
1	tablespoon olive oil
1	(8-ounce) can no-salt-added tomato sauce
3	cups water
1	teaspoon dried rosemary
1	teaspoon salt
1/2	teaspoon black pepper
2	zucchini, cut into 1/2-inch chunks
3	carrots, cut into 1/2-inch chunks
1	onion, cut into chunks
1	teaspoon browning and seasoning sauce

1 Place flour in a shallow dish; add beef chunks and toss to coat completely.

2 In a soup pot over medium-high heat, heat oil. Add beef and sauté 8 to 10 minutes, or until browned on all sides.

3 Add tomato sauce, water, rosemary, salt, and pepper; mix well and bring to a boil. Reduce heat to low, cover, and simmer 1 hour.

4 Add the remaining ingredients, increase heat to high, and return to a boil. Reduce heat to low and simmer 45 to 50 minutes, or until beef and vegetables are tender, stirring occasionally.

Good for You!

Even though the recipe calls for 2 tablespoons of flour, you're going to shake off at least half of that before tossing the coated beef in the oil. This little amount will not only seal in the natural juices in the meat, it will also thicken the stew.

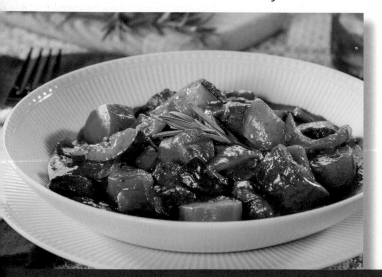

Choices/Exchanges, 3 vegetable, 3 lean protein, 1/2 fat

Calories 230, Calories From Fat 60, **Total Fat** 7.0g, Saturated Fat 2.0g, Trans Fat 0.0g, **Cholesterol** 65mg, **Sodium** 460mg, **Potassium** 660mg, **Total Carbohydrates** 13g, Fiber 3g, Sugar 5g, **Protein** 28g, **Phosphorus** 225mg

Old-World Sausage Stew

Serves 6, about 1-1/2 cups per serving

1	pound turkey sausage, cut into 1/2-inch slices
2	onions, thinly sliced
3	carrots, thinly sliced
3	cups shredded green cabbage
1/2	teaspoon garlic powder
1/2	teaspoon salt (optional)
1/2	teaspoon black pepper
1	cup reduced-sodium chicken broth

1 In a large pot over medium heat, cook turkey sausage, onions, and carrots 8 to 10 minutes, or until sausage is no longer pink, stirring occasionally.

2 Add cabbage, garlic powder, salt, if desired, and pepper, and cook 3 to 4 minutes, stirring occasionally. Add broth and bring to a boil.

3 Reduce heat to low and simmer 6 to 8 minutes, or until cabbage is tender.

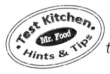

Just so there's no confusion here, this recipe uses raw turkey sausage, not the kind that's already smoked.

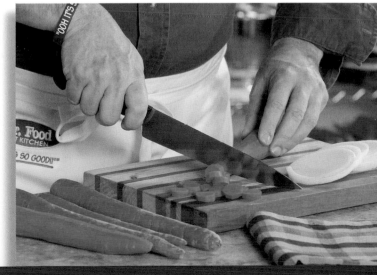

Choices/Exchanges, 2 vegetable, 2 lean protein, 1/2 fat

Calories 160, Calories From Fat 60, **Total Fat** 7.0g, Saturated Fat 1.5g, Trans Fat 0.0g, **Cholesterol** 50mg, **Sodium** 590mg, **Potassium** 460mg, **Total Carbohydrates** 11g, Dietary Fiber 3g, Sugar 5g, **Protein** 15g, **Phosphorus** 175mg

Turkey & 3-Bean Chili

Serves 8, about 1-1/4 cups per serving

1	tablespoon canola oil
1	pound Italian turkey sausage, casing removed
1-1/2	cups chopped onion
1	(15.5 ounce) can no-salt-added black beans, drained
1	(15.5 ounce) can no-salt-added kidney beans, undrained
1	(15.5 ounce) can no-salt-added pinto beans, undrained
1	cup reduced-sodium beef broth
1	cup frozen corn
3/4	cup picante sauce
1	green bell pepper, cut into 3/4-inch pieces
1	red bell pepper, cut into 3/4-inch pieces
1 to 2	drops hot sauce

1 In a large saucepan or Dutch oven, over medium-high heat, heat oil. Break up the sausage and sauté with onion until sausage is browned and onion is tender; drain. Add the remaining ingredients and bring to a boil.

2 Reduce heat to low and simmer, uncovered, 20 minutes, stirring occasionally. Serve immediately.

Good for You!
We love our beef and pork, but did you know that turkey sausage traditionally has less than half of the fat and calories of classic sausage? So it's a natural choice for dishes like this.

Choices/Exchanges, 2 starch, 2 lean protein, 1/2 fat

Calories 280, Calories From Fat 60, **Total Fat** 7.0g, Saturated Fat 1.5g, Trans Fat 0.0g, **Cholesterol** 45mg, **Sodium** 530mg, **Potassium** 270mg, **Total Carbohydrates** 33g, Fiber 9g, Sugar 5g, **Protein** 20g, **Phosphorus** 120mg

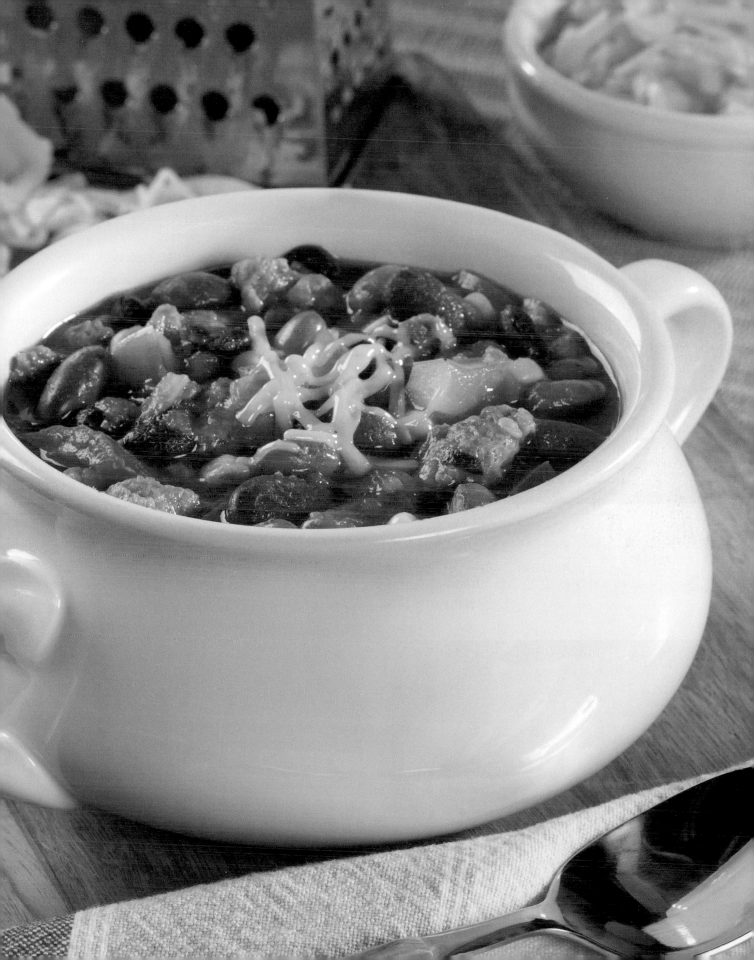

Chunky Texas Chili

Serves 4, about 1-1/2 cups per serving

1	pound boneless bottom round steak, well trimmed and cut into 1/2-inch pieces
1	onion, cut into 1/2-inch chunks
3	garlic cloves, minced
1	(14.5-ounce) can reduced-sodium diced tomatoes, undrained
1-3/4	cups reduced-sodium beef broth
1	(4-ounce) can chopped green chilies, undrained
1	teaspoon cumin
1	teaspoon chili powder
1	teaspoon salt (optional)
1/2	teaspoon black pepper

1 In a soup pot that has been coated with cooking spray, cook the beef, onion, and garlic over medium heat about 10 minutes, or until browned.

2 Add the remaining ingredients, mix well, and bring to a boil. Reduce heat to low and simmer 20 to 25 minutes, or until meat is fork-tender.

Did You Know?

No self-respecting Texan would EVER add beans to chili! It's just tradition! But feel free to garnish with a bit of reduced-fat sour cream and sliced jalapeño if ya feel like dressing it up.

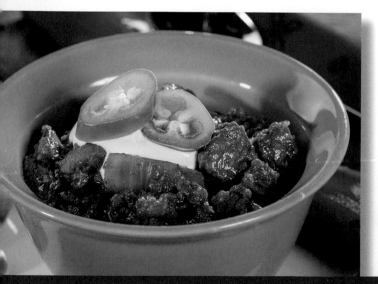

Choices/Exchanges, 2 vegetable, 3 lean protein, 1/2 fat

Calories 220, Calories From Fat 60, **Total Fat** 7.0g, Saturated Fat 2.0g, Trans Fat 0.0g, **Cholesterol** 65mg, **Sodium** 370mg, **Potassium** 760mg, **Total Carbohydrates** 11g, Fiber 2g, Sugar 5g, **Protein** 28g, **Phosphorus** 280mg

Pleasing Poultry

Comforting Chicken Casserole

Serves 6, 1 cup per serving

1	tablespoon canola oil
1	cup chopped red bell pepper
1	cup diced celery
1-1/2	pounds boneless, skinless chicken breast cutlets, cut into 1-inch pieces
1	(10.75-ounce) can reduced-fat, reduced-sodium condensed cream of chicken soup
2/3	cup reduced-fat shredded Cheddar cheese
1	(6-ounce) container fat-free plain yogurt
1/4	cup sliced scallions
1/4	teaspoon black pepper
1/2	cup crushed cornflakes
1/4	cup slivered almonds

1 Preheat oven to 400°F. Lightly coat a 2-quart baking dish with cooking spray.

2 In a large skillet over medium heat, heat oil. Add bell pepper and celery and sauté 3 to 4 minutes, or until tender. Add chicken and continue cooking 5 to 6 minutes, or until chicken is no longer pink. Drain off excess liquid. Stir in soup, cheese, yogurt, scallions, and black pepper. Spoon into prepared baking dish.

3 In a small bowl, combine cornflakes and almonds. Sprinkle evenly over chicken mixture.

4 Bake about 30 minutes, or until heated through.

Good for You!
Fat-free plain yogurt has only 80 calories per 6 ounces and gives recipes a tangy flavor and creamy texture. It's a great substitute for almost anything that calls for mayo.

Choices/Exchanges, 1 carbohydrate, 4 lean protein, 1/2 fat

Calories 280, Calories From Fat 90, **Total Fat** 10.0g, Saturated Fat 2.5g, Trans Fat 0.0g, **Cholesterol** 75mg, **Sodium** 510mg, **Potassium** 700mg, **Total Carbohydrates** 14g, Fiber 2g, Sugar 5g, **Protein** 33g, **Phosphorus** 420mg

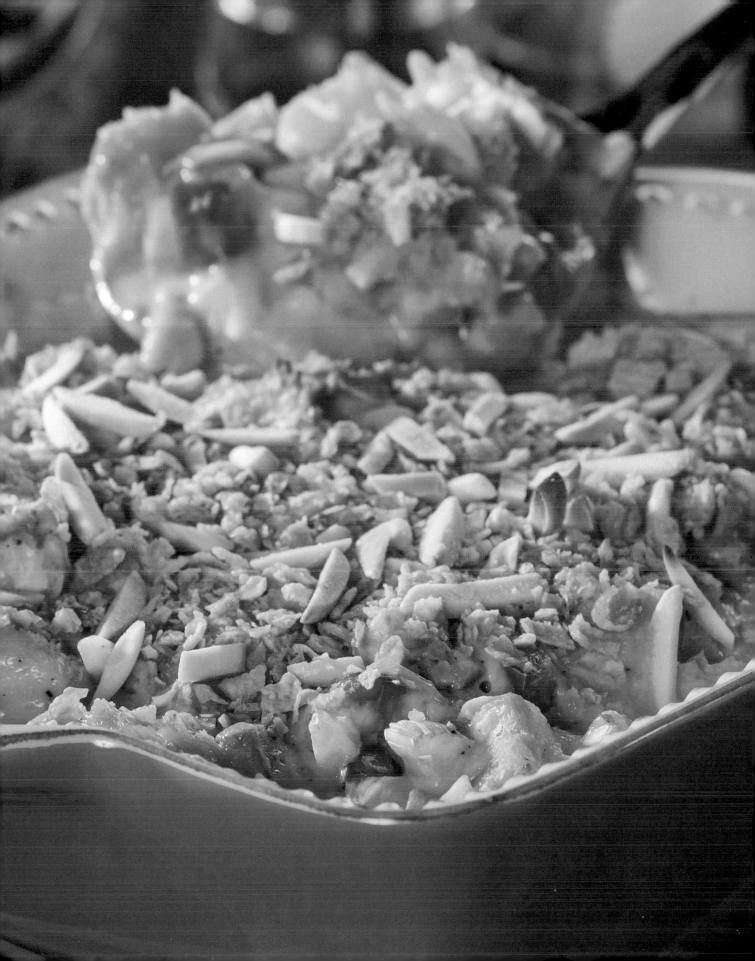

Chicken & Veggie One-Pot

Serves 5, 1-1/4 cups per serving

1	tablespoon olive oil
1	onion, chopped
2	stalks celery, chopped
2	cloves garlic, chopped
1-1/4	pounds boneless, skinless chicken breast cutlets, cut into 1-inch chunks
1/4	pound fresh mushrooms, sliced
2	tablespoons all-purpose flour
1-1/2	cups low-fat milk
1	cup reduced-sodium chicken broth
2	cups cooked brown rice
1/4	cup chopped roasted red peppers
1	cup frozen peas, thawed
1/2	teaspoon dried thyme
1/4	teaspoon salt
1/4	teaspoon black pepper

1 In a large skillet over medium heat, heat oil. Add onion, celery, and garlic, and sauté 3 to 5 minutes, or until tender.

2 Add chicken and mushrooms and sauté 5 minutes, or until chicken is browned. Sprinkle with flour and stir 1 minute, or until absorbed.

3 Add milk and broth and cook 5 to 6 minutes, or until chicken is tender and sauce is thickened, stirring occasionally.

4 Stir in rice, roasted red peppers, peas, thyme, salt, and pepper, and cook 3 to 4 minutes, or until heated through. Serve immediately.

Did You Know?
Brown rice has almost six times the fiber of white rice, and it helps balance your glycemic index. All that, plus it has a rich, nutty taste that really grows on you.

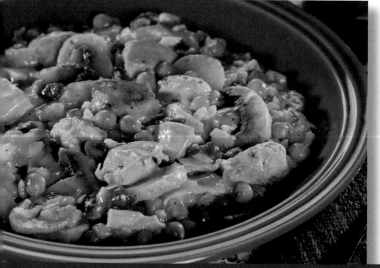

Choices/Exchanges, 2 starch, 1 vegetable, 3 lean protein

Calories 330, Calories From Fat 60, **Total Fat** 7.0g, Saturated Fat 2.0g, Trans Fat 0.0g, **Cholesterol** 70mg, **Sodium** 370mg, **Potassium** 600mg, **Total Carbohydrates** 33g, Fiber 4g, Sugar 8g, **Protein** 31g, **Phosphorus** 375mg

Mexi-Chicken Pizzas

Serves 4, 1 pizza per serving

1/4	cup fat-free sour cream
1	tablespoon fat-free milk
1/4	teaspoon cumin
3	(4-ounce) boneless, skinless chicken breast cutlets, grilled and cut into 1/2-inch pieces
1/4	cup refrigerated fresh salsa
2	whole-wheat pita bread rounds, split horizontally
1	teaspoon olive oil
3/4	cup (3 ounces) reduced-fat shredded sharp Cheddar cheese
1-1/2	cups shredded lettuce
2/3	cup chopped tomatoes
1	tablespoon sliced black olives, drained

1 Preheat oven to 425°F.

2 In a small bowl, mix sour cream, milk, and cumin until well combined; set aside.

3 In another bowl, mix chicken and salsa; set aside.

4 Place pita bread split-side up on a baking sheet. Lightly brush with oil and bake 4 minutes, or until slightly crisp. Spoon chicken mixture evenly over pitas. Sprinkle with cheese.

5 Bake about 5 minutes more, or until chicken is heated through and cheese is melted. Top with lettuce, tomato, and olives. Drizzle with sour cream mixture and serve.

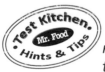

Want a secret way of neatly drizzling the sour cream topping? Spoon mixture into a small, resealable plastic bag, snip off a tiny piece of the corner, and squeeze the topping over pizzas just like a pro!

Choices/Exchanges, 1/2 starch, 1 vegetable, 3 lean protein, 1/2 fat

Calories 220, Calories From Fat 50, **Total Fat** 6.0g, Saturated Fat 2.5g, Trans Fat 0.0g, **Cholesterol** 60mg, **Sodium** 560mg, **Potassium** 460mg, **Total Carbohydrates** 15g, Fiber 2g, Sugar 4g, **Protein** 26g, **Phosphorus** 400mg

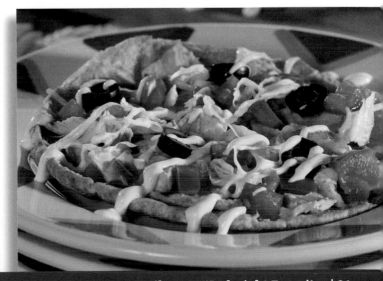

Chicken Fiesta Packets

Serves 4, 1 packet per serving

4	(4-ounce) boneless, skinless chicken breast cutlets
1	tablespoon oil from sun-dried tomatoes
1/2	teaspoon garlic powder
1/2	teaspoon black pepper
1/3	cup thinly sliced sun-dried tomatoes in oil
1/2	cup drained diced green chilies
1	cup frozen corn, thawed

1 Preheat oven to 450°F.

2 Cut 4 (12-inch) squares of aluminum foil. Fold squares in half diagonally, then open squares and lay each cutlet to one side of diagonal crease on each piece of foil.

3 Rub chicken with oil, then sprinkle evenly with garlic powder and pepper. Evenly divide tomatoes, chilies, and corn over chicken cutlets. Loosely fold foil over chicken and seal edges; place packets on a baking sheet.

4 Bake 15 to 18 minutes, checking chicken for doneness. (Be careful when opening the foil packets as the steam could burn you.) If chicken is still pink, reseal and bake 5 additional minutes, or until chicken is no longer pink.

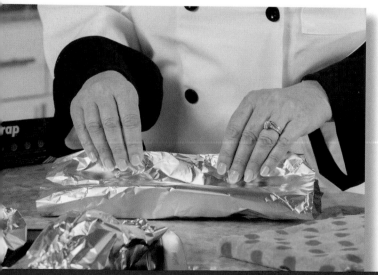

Did You Know?
Chicken breast cutlets can go from juicy to dried out in just seconds if you overcook them. Cooking them in foil helps keep them nice and juicy.

Choices/Exchanges, 1/2 carbohydrate, 3 lean protein

Calories 170, Calories From Fat 25, **Total Fat** 3.0g, Saturated Fat 0.5g, Trans Fat 0.0g, **Cholesterol** 65mg, **Sodium** 170mg, **Potassium** 500mg, **Total Carbohydrates** 8g, Fiber 1g, Sugar <1g, **Protein** 27g, **Phosphorus** 255mg

Parmesan-Crusted Chicken

Serves 4, 1 cutlet per serving

2	tablespoons Dijon mustard
1/2	teaspoon salt (optional)
1/8	teaspoon cayenne pepper
4	(4-ounce) boneless, skinless chicken breast cutlets
1/2	cup reduced-fat grated Parmesan cheese
1/2	cup panko bread crumbs
1	tablespoon chopped parsley
1	teaspoon garlic powder
	Cooking spray

1 Preheat oven to 425°F. Lightly coat a baking sheet with cooking spray.

2 In a large bowl, mix mustard, salt, if desired, and cayenne pepper. Add chicken and turn to coat completely; set aside.

3 In a resealable plastic bag, combine Parmesan cheese, bread crumbs, parsley, and garlic powder. Transfer chicken to bag and shake to coat completely, pressing mixture onto chicken.

4 Place chicken on prepared baking sheet and lightly coat with cooking spray.

5 Bake 15 to 20 minutes, or until cooked through. Serve immediately.

Choices/Exchanges, 1 1/2 starch, 4 lean protein

Calories 290, Calories From Fat 50, **Total Fat** 6.0g, Saturated Fat 2.0g, Trans Fat 0.0g, **Cholesterol** 80mg, **Sodium** 430mg, **Potassium** 390mg, **Total Carbohydrates** 21g, Fiber 0g, Sugar <1g, **Protein** 38g, **Phosphorus** 280mg

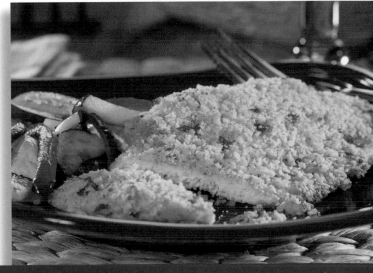

Grilled French Chicken Skewers

Serves 6, 1 skewer per serving

1/4	cup olive oil
1/2	cup balsamic vinegar
2	tablespoons chopped fresh parsley
1	teaspoon dried sage
1	teaspoon dried thyme
3	cloves garlic, minced
1/8	teaspoon salt
1/8	teaspoon black pepper
1-1/2	pounds boneless, skinless chicken breast cutlets, cut into 2-inch strips

1 In a blender, combine oil, vinegar, parsley, sage, thyme, garlic, salt, and pepper; blend well.

2 Place chicken in a resealable plastic bag and pour marinade into bag. Make sure chicken is coated completely and place in refrigerator for at least 2 hours.

3 Preheat grill to medium-high heat. Remove chicken from bag and thread pieces onto six metal skewers. Discard remaining marinade.

4 Grill 8 to 10 minutes, or until chicken is cooked through, turning occasionally.

Serving Suggestion
How about grilling up some zucchini and summer squash to serve with these? Yummy!

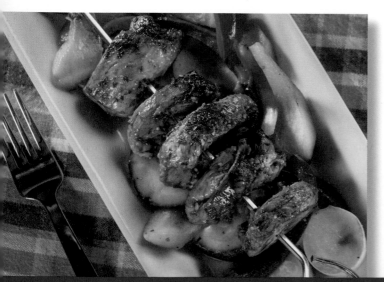

Choices/Exchanges, 4 lean protein, 1 fat

Calories 210, Calories From Fat 90, **Total Fat** 10.0g, Saturated Fat 1.5g, Trans Fat 0.0g, **Cholesterol** 65mg, **Sodium** 125mg, **Potassium** 330mg, **Total Carbohydrates** 2g, Fiber 0g, Sugar 0g, **Protein** 26g, **Phosphorus** 225mg

Greek Isles Chicken

Serves 6, 1 cutlet per serving

2	teaspoons olive oil
6	(4-ounce) boneless, skinless chicken breast cutlets
3	cloves garlic, minced
1/2	cup diced onion
3	tomatoes, diced
1/2	cup reduced-sodium chicken broth
1/2	cup kalamata olives, coarsely chopped
1/2	teaspoon dried oregano
1/4	cup chopped fresh parsley
1/8	teaspoon salt
1/8	teaspoon black pepper
1/4	cup reduced-fat feta cheese crumbles

1. In a large skillet over medium heat, heat oil. Add chicken and sauté 4 to 6 minutes, or until golden, turning once during cooking. Remove chicken to a plate and set aside.

2. Add garlic and onion to skillet and sauté 3 to 4 minutes. Add tomatoes and broth; bring to a boil, then reduce heat to low and simmer 5 minutes.

3. Return chicken to skillet. Add olives, oregano, parsley, salt, and pepper, and cook 2 to 3 minutes, or until warmed through. Sprinkle with feta cheese and serve.

Serving Suggestion

Serve this with a wedge of fresh lemon. Right before digging in, squeeze on the lemon and get ready for a dish that shouts Mediterranean freshness.

Choices/Exchanges, 1 vegetable, 4 lean protein

Calories 220, Calories From Fat 80, **Total Fat** 9.0g, Saturated Fat 1.5g, Trans Fat 0.0g, **Cholesterol** 70mg, **Sodium** 470mg, **Potassium** 510mg, **Total Carbohydrates** 6g, Fiber 1g, Sugar 2g, **Protein** 29g, **Phosphorus** 250mg

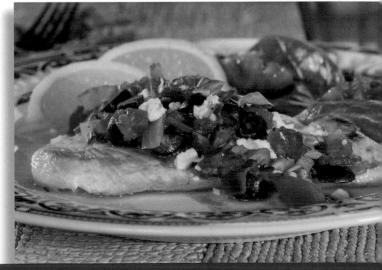

Spinach & Mushroom Chicken Rolls

Serves 4, 1 roll per serving

1/2	cup finely chopped mushrooms
1/2	(10-ounce) package frozen chopped spinach, thawed and squeezed dry
4	ounces fat-free cream cheese, softened
1/2	teaspoon nutmeg
1/2	teaspoon black pepper
4	(4-ounce) boneless, skinless chicken breast cutlets
2	tablespoons reduced-fat shredded Parmesan cheese
2	tablespoons bread crumbs
1/4	teaspoon paprika
	Cooking spray

1 Preheat oven to 350°F.

2 Coat a skillet with cooking spray. Over medium heat, sauté mushrooms 2 to 3 minutes, or until softened, stirring occasionally.

3 Transfer mushrooms to a medium bowl and add spinach, cream cheese, nutmeg, and pepper; mix well. Spoon 2 tablespoons mixture over each chicken cutlet. Roll up and secure with toothpicks. Place rolls in a 9 × 13-inch baking dish.

4 In a small bowl, mix Parmesan cheese, bread crumbs, and paprika. Sprinkle mixture evenly over chicken and lightly coat with cooking spray.

5 Bake rolls 25 to 30 minutes, or until no pink remains in chicken.

Serving Suggestion

Try serving these with some steamed green beans accented with red peppers. Not only do they add color to the plate, they're the perfect, healthy go-along.

Choices/Exchanges, 1/2 carbohydrate, 4 lean protein

Calories 200, Calories From Fat 30, **Total Fat** 3.5g, Saturated Fat 1.0g, Trans Fat 0.0g, **Cholesterol** 70mg, **Sodium** 330mg, **Potassium** 510mg, **Total Carbohydrates** 8g, Fiber 2g, Sugar <1g, **Protein** 33g, **Phosphorus** 380mg

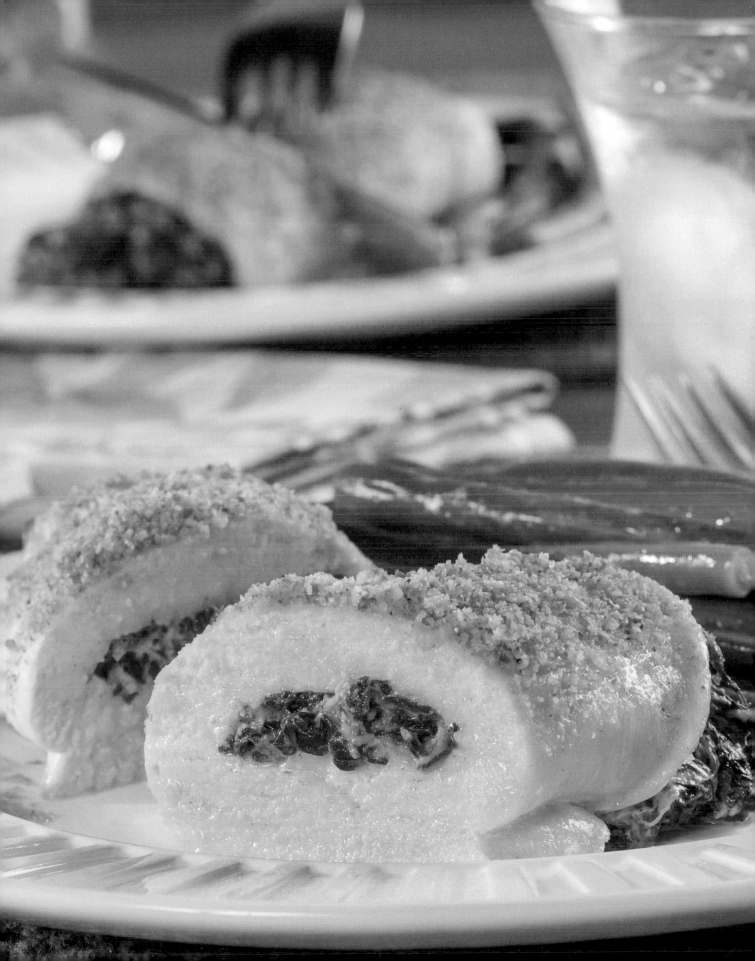

Citrus-Glazed Chicken

Serves 4, 2 pieces per serving

1	(3-pound) chicken, cut into 8 pieces, skin removed
1/2	teaspoon salt
1/2	cup sugar-free orange marmalade
1	(11-ounce) can mandarin oranges, drained
1	green bell pepper, seeded and cut into 1-inch pieces
1	tablespoon lemon juice
1/8	teaspoon cayenne pepper

1 Preheat oven to 400°F. Coat a 9 × 13-inch baking dish with cooking spray.

2 Place chicken in prepared baking dish. Season with salt.

3 Bake 35 minutes; drain off excess liquid.

4 In a bowl, combine the remaining ingredients and pour over chicken.

5 Bake 20 to 25 minutes longer, or until chicken is no longer pink and juices run clear.

Good for You!
Did you know that by removing the skin of the chicken we save 3.5 grams of saturated fat and 90 calories per serving? See, it's little things like this that make the difference.

Choices/Exchanges, 1 carbohydrate, 4 lean protein

Calories 260, Calories From Fat 70, **Total Fat** 8.0g, Saturated Fat 2.5g, Trans Fat 0.0g, **Cholesterol** 95mg, **Sodium** 390mg, **Potassium** 420mg, **Total Carbohydrates** 11g, Fiber 1g, Sugar 5g, **Protein** 32g, **Phosphorus** 230mg

Chicken & Broccoli "Spaghetti" Squash

Serves 4, 2 cups per serving

1	whole spaghetti squash (yields about 5 cups of strands)
2	tablespoons olive oil
4	cloves garlic, minced
1	cup low-sodium chicken broth, divided
1/3	cup chopped sun-dried tomatoes (not in oil)
2	cups broccoli florets
4	(4-ounce) boneless, skinless chicken breast cutlets, grilled and cut into 1/2-inch strips
1/4	cup grated Parmesan cheese
1/8	teaspoon black pepper
1	teaspoon pine nuts

1 Fill a soup pot with 1 inch water and place whole squash in pot. Bring to a boil over high heat, cover, and cook 20 to 30 minutes, or until squash is tender when pierced with a knife. Remove to a cutting board and allow to cool slightly. Cut squash in half lengthwise, then use a spoon to remove and discard seeds. Scrape inside of squash with a fork, shredding into noodle-like strands; set aside.

2 In a large, deep skillet, over medium-high heat, heat oil. Add garlic and sauté 1 minute. Add 1/4 cup broth, sun-dried tomatoes, and broccoli, and cook 5 minutes.

3 Add chicken, remaining broth, Parmesan cheese, and pepper. Reduce heat to medium-low and simmer about 3 minutes, or until heated through.

4 Spoon chicken mixture over spaghetti squash, sprinkle with pine nuts, and serve.

Did You Know?
It takes about 5 pounds of fresh tomatoes to make 2 cups of sun-dried tomatoes. Who would have ever imagined?

Choices/Exchanges, 4 vegetable, 4 lean protein, 1/2 fat

Calories 300, Calories From Fat 110, **Total Fat** 12.0g, Saturated Fat 2.5g, Trans Fat 0.0g, **Cholesterol** 70mg, **Sodium** 330mg, **Potassium** 860mg, **Total Carbohydrates** 19g, Fiber 3g, Sugar 7g, **Protein** 33g, **Phosphorus** 360mg

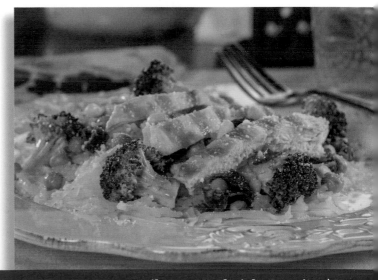

Chinatown Chicken Salad

Serves 6, 2 cups per serving

Dressing

1/4	cup sesame oil
1/4	cup rice vinegar
2	cloves garlic, minced
2	tablespoons sugar
2	tablespoons low-sodium soy sauce
2	tablespoons ground ginger
1	tablespoon canola oil
2	teaspoons prepared yellow mustard

Salad

1	pound boneless, skinless chicken breast cutlets
1	head Napa cabbage, shredded
2	carrots, shredded
3	scallions, sliced
1/2	cup cilantro leaves, coarsely chopped
1/2	cup slivered almonds

1 In a jar or plastic container with a tight-fitting lid, combine all the dressing ingredients and shake well.

2 Pour half the dressing into a large, resealable plastic bag and refrigerate remaining dressing. Add chicken to plastic bag; seal bag and shake to coat. Refrigerate at least 30 minutes.

3 Heat a grill pan or skillet over medium heat. Remove chicken from marinade and place in pan. Discard excess marinade. Cook chicken 8 to 10 minutes, or until no longer pink, turning halfway through cooking; let cool. Cut chicken into bite-sized pieces and set aside.

4 In a large bowl, place cabbage, carrots, scallions, cilantro, almonds, and chicken. Before serving, drizzle with remaining dressing and toss.

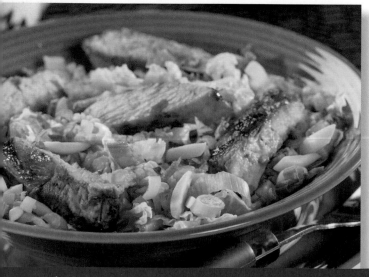

Choices/Exchanges, 1/2 carbohydrate, 2 vegetable, 2 lean protein, 3 fat

Calories 320, Calories From Fat 170, **Total Fat** 19.0g, Saturated Fat 2.0g, Trans Fat 0.0g, **Cholesterol** 45mg, **Sodium** 300mg, **Potassium** 520mg, **Total Carbohydrates** 19g, Fiber 3g, Sugar 6g, **Protein** 21g, **Phosphorus** 230mg

Italian Stuffed Zucchini

Serves 4, 2 stuffed zucchini halves per serving

4	large zucchini
3/4	pound ground turkey breast
1/4	pound Italian turkey sausage, casing removed
1	(14.5-ounce) can no-salt-added diced tomatoes, drained
1/2	cup (2 ounces) reduced-fat shredded mozzarella cheese, divided
1/2	teaspoon Italian seasoning
1/8	teaspoon salt

1 Preheat oven to 350°F.

2 Cut each zucchini in half lengthwise and scoop out the flesh, leaving a 1/4-inch shell. Dice flesh that was removed.

3 In a large skillet over medium heat, cook ground turkey, sausage, and diced zucchini 5 minutes, or until cooked through, breaking up turkey and turkey sausage with a spoon while cooking. Drain mixture and place in a bowl. Add tomatoes, 1/4 cup mozzarella cheese, Italian seasoning, and salt; mix well.

4 Fill zucchini halves with mixture and place on a rimmed baking sheet.

5 Bake 20 minutes; remove from oven, and sprinkle with remaining cheese. Bake 5 more minutes, or until cheese is melted and filling is heated through. Serve immediately.

Test Kitchen. Mr. Food Hints & Tips

To scoop out the inside of the zucchini, simply take a soup spoon and scrape it down the middle of each half. The fleshy part will easily scoop right out.

Choices/Exchanges, 2 vegetable, 4 lean protein

Calories 230, Calories From Fat 60, **Total Fat** 7.0g, Saturated Fat 2.0g, Trans Fat 0.0g, **Cholesterol** 60mg, **Sodium** 450mg, **Potassium** 760mg, **Total Carbohydrates** 12g, Fiber 3g, Sugar 7g, **Protein** 32g, **Phosphorus** 185mg

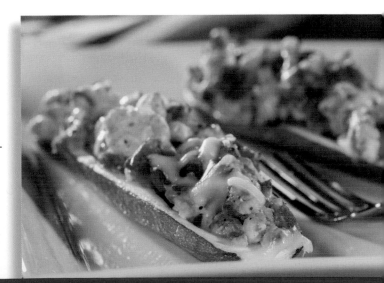

Broccoli & Cheese Turkey Rollups

Serves 6, 1 rollup per serving

1	(16-ounce) package frozen chopped broccoli, thawed
1/2	cup (2-ounces) fat-free shredded sharp Cheddar cheese
3/4	cup whole-wheat bread crumbs, divided
1/2	teaspoon onion powder
1/4	teaspoon black pepper
6	(4-ounce) boneless, skinless turkey breast cutlets
1	(10.75-ounce) can fat-free broccoli cheese soup

1 Preheat oven to 350°F. Coat a 9 × 13-inch baking dish with cooking spray.

2 In a large bowl, combine broccoli, cheese, 1/2 cup bread crumbs, onion powder, and pepper; mix well.

3 Place turkey cutlets on a cutting board and place an equal amount of the stuffing mixture in center of each cutlet. Roll up cutlets and place seam-side down in prepared baking dish. Spoon soup evenly over top of cutlets and sprinkle with remaining bread crumbs.

4 Cover and bake 35 to 40 minutes, or until cooked through and no pink remains in the turkey.

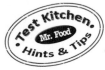

Test Kitchen. Mr. Food Hints & Tips

If you don't see turkey cutlets in the meat case, simply ask the butcher. They'll likely be happy to cut some fresh for you.

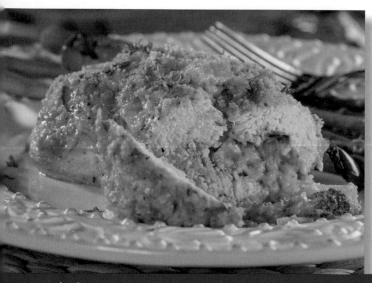

Choices/Exchanges, 2 carbohydrate, 2 lean protein

Calories 230, Calories From Fat 25, **Total Fat** 3.0g, Saturated Fat 0.5g, Trans Fat 0.0g, **Cholesterol** 15mg, **Sodium** 570mg, **Potassium** 650mg, **Total Carbohydrates** 33g, Fiber 6g, Sugar 4g, **Protein** 15g, **Phosphorus** 220mg

Corn Muffin Sloppy Joes

Serves 4, 1 Sloppy Joe per serving

1/2	pound ground turkey breast
1	cup frozen pepper stir-fry (sliced green, red, and yellow bell peppers and white onions)
1/4	cup no-salt-added tomato sauce
1/4	cup reduced-sodium barbecue sauce
1/4	cup water
1/2	teaspoon garlic powder
1	teaspoon chili powder
1/2	teaspoon cumin
4	corn muffins (2-1/2 × 2-1/2-inch)

1 Coat a large, nonstick skillet with cooking spray. Over medium heat, cook turkey until browned, breaking up meat with a spoon while cooking. Remove from skillet and set aside.

2 In the same skillet, cook pepper and onion mixture until lightly browned. Return turkey to skillet and add tomato sauce, barbecue sauce, water, garlic powder, chili powder, and cumin. Simmer about 8 minutes, or until heated through, adding additional water if you prefer a looser consistency.

3 Meanwhile, split corn muffins crosswise and toast. Place muffin bottoms on plates. Top with sloppy Joe mixture and muffin tops; serve.

Did You Know?
Frozen vegetables are picked at their nutritional and flavor peak, then flash frozen to lock in their color, nutrition, and taste. So they are often fresher than fresh veggies.

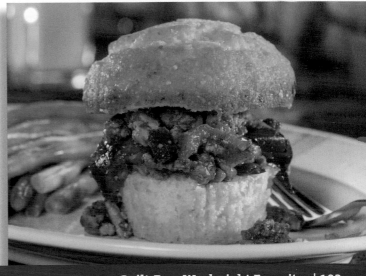

Choices/Exchanges, 2 starch, 1/2 carbohydrate, 2 lean protein

Calories 280, Calories From Fat 45, **Total Fat** 5.0g, Saturated Fat 1.0g, Trans Fat 0.0g, **Cholesterol** 65mg, **Sodium** 590mg, **Potassium** 360mg, **Total Carbohydrates** 39g, Fiber 3g, Sugar 11g, **Protein** 18g, **Phosphorus** 225mg

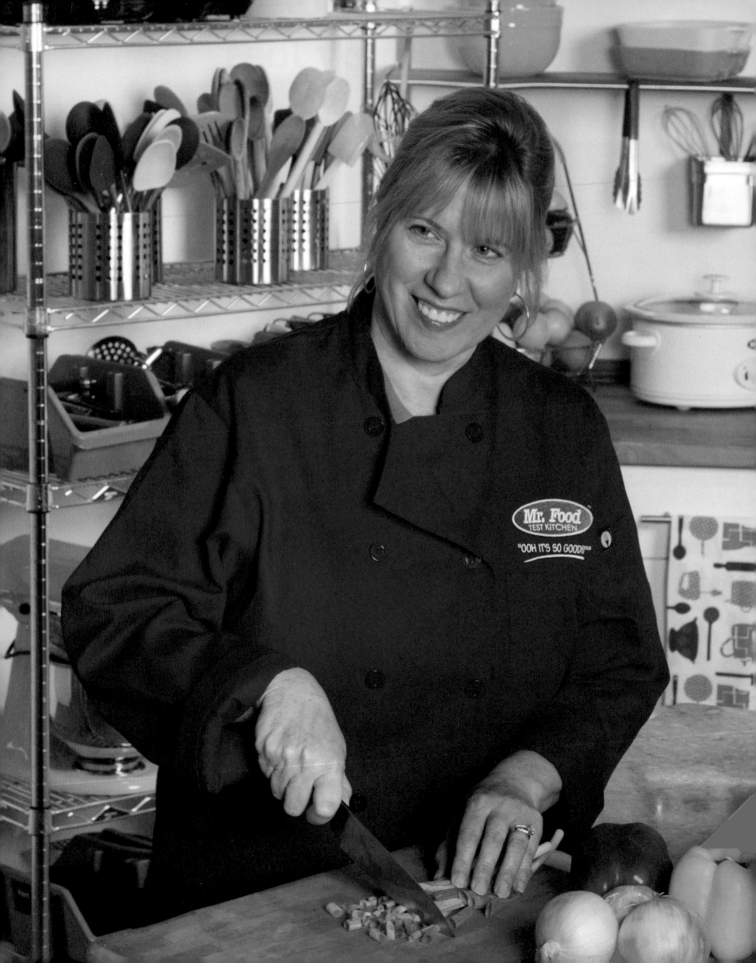

Hearty Beef & Pork

Rancher's Steak with Cowboy Caviar

Serves 6, 1/6 of recipe per serving

1	tablespoon chili powder
1	teaspoon ground cumin
1	teaspoon salt
1/2	teaspoon cayenne pepper
2-1/2	pounds well-trimmed boneless beef top sirloin steak, about 1 inch thick
1	(15-ounce) can black beans, rinsed and drained
1	tomato, seeded and chopped
1/2	red onion, chopped
3	tablespoons coarsely chopped cilantro

1 Preheat the broiler. Coat a rimmed baking sheet with cooking spray.

2 In a small bowl, combine the chili powder, cumin, salt, and cayenne pepper; mix well and set aside 2 teaspoons. Rub the remaining mixture evenly over the entire steak and place on prepared baking sheet.

3 Broil the steak 25 to 30 minutes for medium-rare to medium, or until desired doneness, turning once during the broiling.

4 Meanwhile, make the Cowboy Caviar. In a medium bowl, combine the remaining ingredients, including the reserved seasoning mixture; mix well.

5 Let steak rest 5 minutes before thinly slicing beef across the grain. Serve topped with the Cowboy Caviar.

Test Kitchen, Mr. Food Hints & Tips

We like to make the Cowboy Caviar ahead of time and refrigerate it to allow the flavors to blend well. Then, when you serve the chilled mixture over the warm, sliced steak, get ready for some real hootin' and hollerin'.

Choices/Exchanges, 1 starch, 1 vegetable, 6 lean protein

Calories 350, Calories From Fat 80, **Total Fat** 9.0g, Saturated Fat 3.0g, Trans Fat 0.0g, **Cholesterol** 70mg, **Sodium** 510mg, **Potassium** 1000mg, **Total Carbohydrates** 20g, Fiber 7g, Sugar <1g, **Protein** 47g, **Phosphorus** 495mg

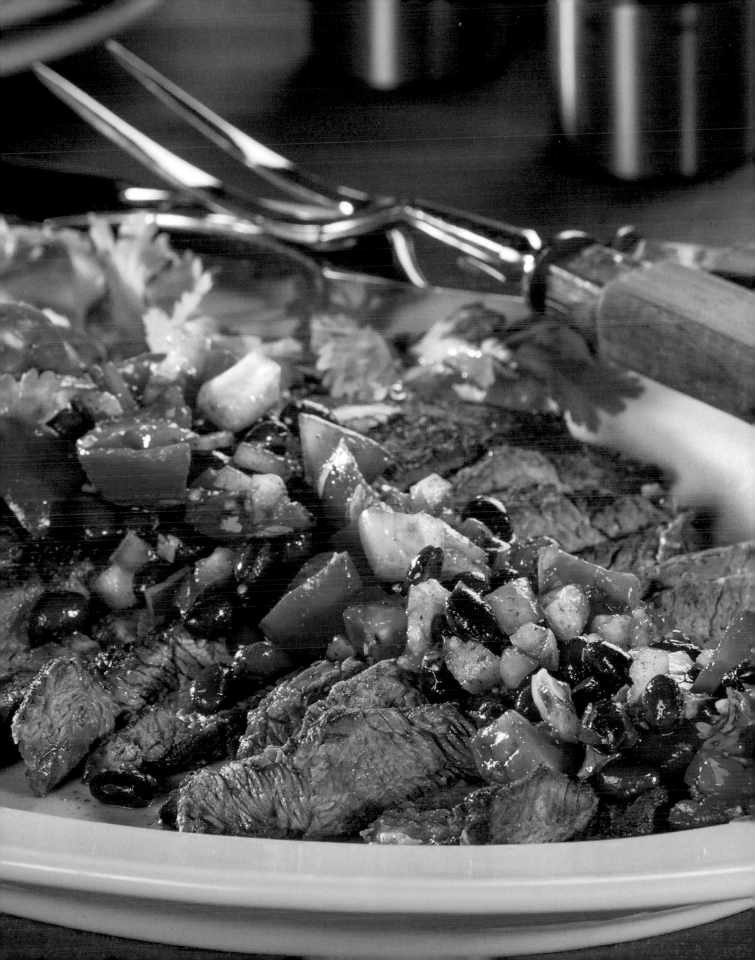

My Momma's Meat Loaf

Serves 8, 1 slice per serving

2	pounds 95% extra-lean ground beef
1/2	green bell pepper, finely chopped
1	onion, finely chopped
1	egg
1	cup rolled oats
1	cup ketchup, divided
1-1/2	teaspoons garlic powder
1/4	teaspoon salt
1/2	teaspoon black pepper
1	tablespoon brown sugar

1 Preheat oven to 350°F. Coat a 9 × 5-inch loaf pan with cooking spray.

2 In a large bowl, combine ground beef, green bell pepper, onion, egg, oats, 3/4 cup ketchup, garlic powder, salt, and pepper. Using your hands, gently mix just until combined. (Try not to over-handle mixture.) Place in prepared pan.

3 Bake 1 hour. Brush with remaining ketchup, sprinkle with brown sugar, and bake 10 to 15 additional minutes, or until no pink remains. Drain any excess liquid, let cool 5 to 10 minutes, then cut into 8 slices and serve.

Just a Thought

If you think this is good hot out of the oven, then you'll love how Momma used to serve it the next day. She would slice it, reheat it in a skillet, and serve it open-faced on a slice of bread with a little ketchup. Yummy!

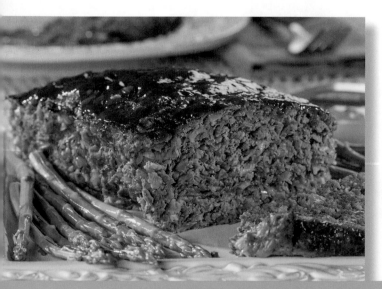

Choices/Exchanges, 1 1/2 carbohydrate, 3 lean protein

Calories 250, Calories From Fat 50, **Total Fat** 6.0g, Saturated Fat 2.5g, Trans Fat 0.0g, **Cholesterol** 80mg, **Sodium** 470mg, **Potassium** 550mg, **Total Carbohydrates** 24g, Fiber 3g, Sugar 9g, **Protein** 23g, **Phosphorus** 130mg

Simple Southern Sliders

Serves 6, 2 sliders per serving

3	tablespoons reduced-fat mayonnaise
4	tablespoons sugar-free peach preserves, divided
1/8	teaspoon plus 1/2 teaspoon salt, divided (optional)
1-1/4	pounds 95% extra-lean ground beef
1	teaspoon onion powder
1/2	teaspoon black pepper
3	ultra-thin slices pepper-jack cheese, each cut into quarters (optional)
1	(12-count) package whole-wheat slider rolls, toasted

1. In a small bowl, combine mayonnaise, 2 tablespoons peach preserves, and 1/8 teaspoon salt, if desired. Mix well and refrigerate until ready to use.

2. Preheat grill to medium-high heat.

3. In a medium bowl, combine ground beef, remaining peach preserves, onion powder, remaining salt, if desired, and pepper; mix well. Divide mixture into 12 equal amounts and form into 12 slider patties.

4. Grill patties 4 to 6 minutes, or until no pink remains, turning them over halfway through grilling.

5. If desired, place a piece of cheese on each slider about 2 minutes before burgers are finished cooking. When done, place each patty on a toasted roll and top with peach mayonnaise.

Did You Know?

Sliders were first introduced to America by White Castle and cost only 5¢ apiece until the 1940s. After that they were 10¢ apiece for the longest time. Boy, those were the good old days.

Choices/Exchanges, 2 1/2 starch, 4 lean protein

Calories 370, Calories From Fat 90, **Total Fat** 10.0g, Saturated Fat 2.5g, Trans Fat 0.0g, **Cholesterol** 60mg, **Sodium** 390mg, **Potassium** 330mg, **Total Carbohydrates** 40g, Fiber 7g, Sugar 7g, **Protein** 34g, **Phosphorus** 190mg

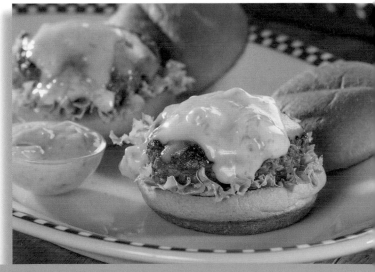

Toasty Roast Beef Wraps

Serves 4, 1 wrap per serving

2	tablespoons fat-free plain Greek yogurt
1	tablespoon honey
1	tablespoon spicy brown mustard
4	(10-inch) whole-wheat tortillas
1/2	pound thinly sliced low-sodium deli roast beef
1/2	cup (2 ounces) fat-free shredded Cheddar cheese
3/4	cup diced tomato
1/2	cup diced red onion

1 Preheat oven to 375°F.

2 In a small bowl, combine yogurt, honey, and mustard.

3 Spread tortillas out on a work surface. Spread 1 tablespoon honey-mustard mixture on each tortilla. Layer evenly with roast beef, then sprinkle evenly with cheese, tomato, and onion.

4 Fold in sides of each tortilla and roll up like a burrito. Wrap each in foil and bake in oven 10 to 15 minutes, or until heated through. Cut each in half and serve.

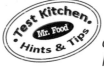

Test Kitchen Mr. Food Hints & Tips

You can make these ahead of time and just pop them in the oven, or even the toaster oven, to warm through whenever you get the hankering for something hearty and cheesy that'll fill ya up.

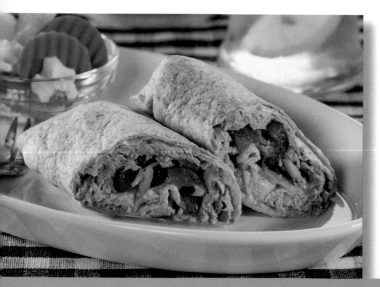

Choices/Exchanges, 2 starch, 2 lean protein, 1/2 fat

Calories 270, Calories From Fat 60, **Total Fat** 7.0g, Saturated Fat 2.5g, Trans Fat 0.0g, **Cholesterol** 35mg, **Sodium** 510mg, **Potassium** 95mg, **Total Carbohydrates** 29g, Fiber 15g, Sugar 6g, **Protein** 23g, **Phosphorus** 40mg

Slow Cooker Pot Roast

Serves 8, 1/8 of recipe per serving

1	teaspoon salt
1/2	teaspoon black pepper
1/2	teaspoon garlic powder
3	pounds well-trimmed boneless beef bottom round roast
1	(16-ounce) package baby carrots
1	large onion, sliced into half moons
1-1/2	cups peeled and cubed sweet potatoes
1-1/2	cups peeled and cubed russet baking potatoes
1	(12-ounce) can diet cola
1	(12-ounce) bottle chili sauce
2	tablespoons Worcestershire sauce
2	tablespoons hot pepper sauce

1 Sprinkle salt, pepper, and garlic powder evenly over entire roast, then place roast in a 6-quart slow cooker. Place carrots, onion, sweet potatoes, and baking potatoes around roast.

2 In a medium bowl, combine the remaining ingredients; mix well, then pour over roast.

3 Cover and cook on HIGH 6 hours or LOW 8 hours, or until fork-tender. Slice and serve topped with sauce and vegetables.

Just a Thought

The beauty of making pot roast in a slow cooker is that it takes a relatively inexpensive cut of meat and turns it into the most tender and flavor-packed roast you've ever tasted. Plus the cola makes this even more tender and gives it a super-rich taste.

Choices/Exchanges, 1 starch, 1/2 carbohydrate, 1 vegetable, 5 lean protein

Calories 350, Calories From Fat 60, **Total Fat** 7.0g, Saturated Fat 2.0g, Trans Fat 0.0g, **Cholesterol** 85mg, **Sodium** 580mg, **Potassium** 1310mg, **Total Carbohydrates** 32g, Fiber 3g, Sugar 14g, **Protein** 41g, **Phosphorus** 445mg

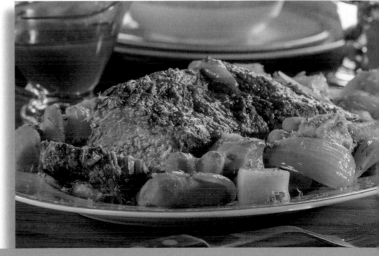

Threaded Churrasco Steak

Serves 8, 4 skewers per serving

3/4	cup olive oil
2	tablespoons lime juice
1/2	cup fresh parsley, stems removed
4	cloves garlic
1	teaspoon chili powder
1/2	teaspoon salt
1/4	teaspoon black pepper
2	pounds well-trimmed boneless beef top sirloin steak, cut into 32 (1/2-inch) strips across the grain
32	(6-inch) skewers

1 In a food processor or blender, combine oil, lime juice, parsley, garlic, chili powder, salt, and pepper; process until marinade is well blended.

2 Thread one piece of steak onto each skewer. Place skewers in a 9 × 13-inch baking dish and pour marinade over steak; cover and refrigerate 1 hour.

3 Heat a grill pan over medium-high heat and cook steak on skewers 2 to 3 minutes per side, or until desired doneness.

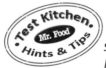

These can be cooked on the grill, too. If you are using wooden skewers, just make sure you soak them in water for a few minutes before skewering the meat to prevent them from burning.

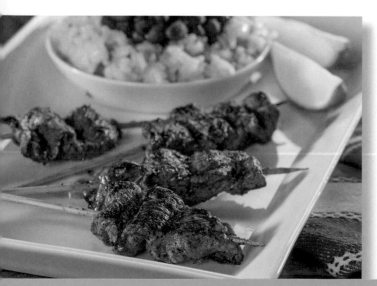

Choices/Exchanges, 3 lean protein, 2 fat

Calories 230, Calories From Fat 130, **Total Fat** 14.0g, Saturated Fat 3.0g, Trans Fat 0.0g, **Cholesterol** 40mg, **Sodium** 210mg, **Potassium** 430mg, **Total Carbohydrates** 1g, Fiber 0g, Sugar 0g, **Protein** 24g, **Phosphorus** 235mg

Meat 'n' Potato Casserole

Serves 6, 1-1/4 cups per serving

1	pound 95% extra-lean ground beef
1	onion, chopped
2	cloves garlic, minced
1	(14.5-ounce) can no-salt-added diced tomatoes, undrained
1	tablespoon chili powder
1/2	teaspoon garlic powder
1/2	teaspoon black pepper
2	cups shredded green cabbage
3	tablespoons salsa
1	small russet baking potato, not peeled, shredded
	Cooking spray
1/4	cup (2 ounces) reduced-fat shredded mozzarella cheese
1	tablespoon reduced-fat grated Parmesan cheese

1 Preheat oven to 375°F. Lightly coat a 2-quart casserole dish with cooking spray.

2 In a large skillet over medium-high heat, brown ground beef, onion, and garlic, breaking up beef with a spoon while cooking. Drain off excess liquid. Stir in tomatoes with their juice, chili powder, garlic powder, pepper, and cabbage. Sauté 1 to 2 minutes, or until heated through, stirring often. Add salsa, stirring to combine.

3 Spoon mixture into prepared casserole dish. Top with potatoes, lightly coat with cooking spray, and bake 30 minutes, or until crisp.

4 Sprinkle with cheeses and bake another 5 minutes, or until cheese is melted. Serve immediately.

Good for You!

When making recipes with potatoes, don't feel that you have to peel them. After all, the skins are loaded with all sorts of vitamins and are a great source of fiber.

Choices/Exchanges, 1 carbohydrate, 2 lean protein, 1/2 fat

Calories 180, Calories From Fat 50, **Total Fat** 6.0g, Saturated Fat 2.5g, Trans Fat 0.0g, **Cholesterol** 50mg, **Sodium** 150mg, **Potassium** 650mg, **Total Carbohydrates** 12g, Fiber 3g, Sugar 5g, **Protein** 20g, **Phosphorus** 220mg

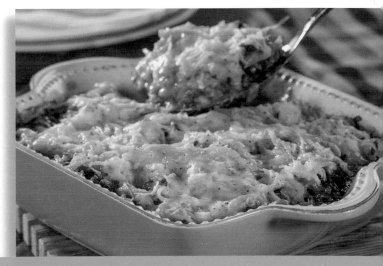

Fancy-Schmancy Beef Tenderloin

Serves 4, 1/4 recipe per serving

1/4	cup balsamic vinegar
3	teaspoons canola oil, divided
1/8	teaspoon crushed red pepper flakes
6	ounces Portobello mushrooms, cut into 1-1/2-inch slices
4	(4-ounce) beef tenderloin steaks, sliced crosswise into medallions
1/4	teaspoon salt
1/2	teaspoon black pepper
1	onion, finely chopped
1/4	cup low-sodium beef broth
1	tablespoon chopped fresh parsley

1. In a resealable plastic bag, combine vinegar, 2 teaspoons oil, and crushed red pepper. Add mushrooms and turn to coat completely. Marinate 15 minutes.

2. Meanwhile, sprinkle medallions with salt and pepper.

3. In a large skillet over medium-high heat, heat remaining oil. Add beef and sauté 2 minutes on each side, or to desired doneness. Place on a serving platter and cover to keep warm.

4. Remove mushrooms from marinade, reserving marinade. In the same skillet, over medium heat, cook mushrooms and onion 3 to 5 minutes, or until softened. Add reserved marinade, broth, and parsley; bring to a boil and cook 1 to 2 minutes, or until sauce begins to thicken. Spoon over beef and serve immediately.

Did You Know?

Beef tenderloin is also known as filet mignon and is often considered the Cadillac of all cuts of beef. It is a bit more expensive, but worth the splurge every once in a while.

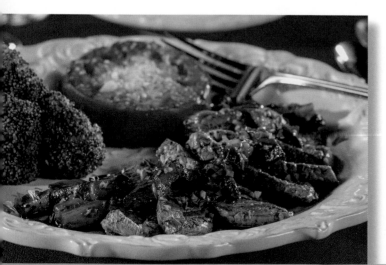

Choices/Exchanges, 1 vegetable, 3 lean protein, 1 fat

Calories 230, Calories From Fat 100, **Total Fat** 11.0g, Saturated Fat 3.0g, Trans Fat 0.0g, **Cholesterol** 70mg, **Sodium** 230mg, **Potassium** 660mg, **Total Carbohydrates** 6g, Fiber 1g, Sugar 2g, **Protein** 26g, **Phosphorus** 300mg

Beef & Broccoli Lo Mein

Serves 4, 1/4 recipe per serving

3	tablespoons low-sodium soy sauce, divided
2	teaspoons sesame oil, divided
1	tablespoon cornstarch
1	pound beef sirloin, well trimmed and thinly sliced
2	tablespoons olive oil, divided
4	garlic cloves, chopped
1	pound broccoli florets
1	red bell pepper, cut into strips
1	red onion, cut in half and thinly sliced
3/4	cup reduced-sodium beef broth
1	teaspoon ground ginger
1	teaspoon granulated Splenda
3/4	pound cooked linguine

1. In a large, resealable plastic bag, combine 1 tablespoon soy sauce, 1 teaspoon sesame oil, and cornstarch. Add beef, and turn to coat completely. Marinate in refrigerator 1 hour.

2. In a large, nonstick skillet over medium heat, heat 1 tablespoon olive oil. Add garlic and cook 1 minute. Add broccoli, bell pepper, and onion, and cook 3 to 5 minutes, or until crisp-tender, stirring frequently. Transfer vegetables to a bowl.

3. In the same skillet, over medium-high heat, heat remaining olive oil. Add beef and cook 4 to 6 minutes, or until no pink remains. Add to vegetables.

4. In the same skillet, over medium-high heat, add remaining soy sauce, remaining sesame oil, broth, ginger, and Splenda. Bring to a boil, scraping up any bits from the pan. Add linguine and cook 2 to 3 minutes, or until liquid is almost completely absorbed. Return beef and vegetables to skillet and toss to combine. Serve immediately.

Did You Know?

"Mein" is the Chinese word for "noodles," and "lo mein" simply means "tossed noodles." See, won't that be a fun little fact to talk about at the dinner table?

Choices/Exchanges, 2 starch, 2 vegetable, 3 lean protein, 2 fat

Calories 440, Calories From Fat 140, **Total Fat** 15.0g, Saturated Fat 3.0g, Trans Fat 0.0g, **Cholesterol** 40mg, **Sodium** 580mg, **Potassium** 890mg, **Total Carbohydrates** 43g, Fiber 6g, Sugar 6g, **Protein** 33g, **Phosphorus** 345mg

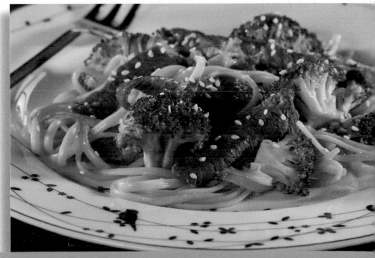

Greek Burgers

Serves 4, 1 burger per serving

Cucumber Sauce

1/2	cup fat-free sour cream
1/2	cup finely diced cucumber
1/2	teaspoon dill weed
1	clove garlic, minced
1	teaspoon lemon juice
1/4	teaspoon salt
1/8	teaspoon black pepper

Burgers

3/4	pound 95% extra-lean ground beef
1	cup cooked brown rice
1/2	teaspoon onion powder
1/2	teaspoon garlic powder
1	teaspoon oregano
1/4	teaspoon salt
1/4	teaspoon black pepper
1/4	cup fat-free feta crumbles

1. In a small bowl, combine Cucumber Sauce ingredients; set aside.

2. In a large bowl, combine the remaining ingredients; mix well. Divide into 4 patties.

3. Coat a grill pan or large skillet with cooking spray. Cook burgers over medium heat 4 to 5 minutes per side, or until no pink remains.

4. Serve burgers topped with Cucumber Sauce.

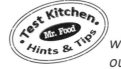

When the weather is nice, these will also grill up great on your outdoor grill. So year-round you can say, like they do in Greece … OPA!!

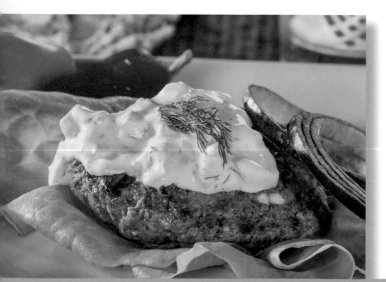

Choices/Exchanges, 1 carbohydrate, 3 lean protein

Calories 220, Calories From Fat 45, **Total Fat** 5.0g, Saturated Fat 2.0g, Trans Fat 0.0g, **Cholesterol** 55mg, **Sodium** 490mg, **Potassium** 480mg, **Total Carbohydrates** 19g, Fiber 1g, Sugar 3g, **Protein** 23g, **Phosphorus** 80mg

Beefy Enchiladas

Serves 4, 1 enchilada per serving

1	cup chunky picante sauce, divided
1/2	red bell pepper, diced
1/2	green bell pepper, diced
1/4	cup chopped onion
1/2	pound 95% extra-lean ground beef
1	teaspoon cumin
1	teaspoon chili powder
1/2	teaspoon garlic powder
1/2	cup (2 ounces) reduced-fat shredded Mexican cheese blend, divided
4	(6-inch) corn tortillas
2	tablespoons chopped fresh cilantro

1 Preheat oven to 400°F. In a 9-inch square baking dish, spread 1/4 cup picante sauce; set aside.

2 In a large skillet over medium-high heat, sauté bell peppers, onion, and ground beef until peppers are soft and beef is browned. Drain excess liquid. Stir in 1/2 cup picante sauce, cumin, chili powder, and garlic powder, and simmer 5 minutes, stirring occasionally. Remove from heat; stir in half the cheese.

3 Stack the tortillas and wrap in wax paper. Heat in microwave on HIGH 10 seconds, or until warmed.

4 Spoon 1/2 cup meat mixture down center of each tortilla. Top evenly with remaining picante sauce, remaining cheese, and the cilantro. Roll up and serve.

Did You Know?
In Mexico, enchiladas are considered street/fast food, are bought wrapped in foil, and eaten much like we do our hot dogs.

Choices/Exchanges, 1 starch, 1 vegetable, 2 lean protein

Calories 190, Calories From Fat 45, **Total Fat** 5.0g, Saturated Fat 2.0g, Trans Fat 0.0g, **Cholesterol** 40mg, **Sodium** 480mg, **Potassium** 490mg, **Total Carbohydrates** 20g, Fiber 3g, Sugar 5g, **Protein** 17g, **Phosphorus** 305mg

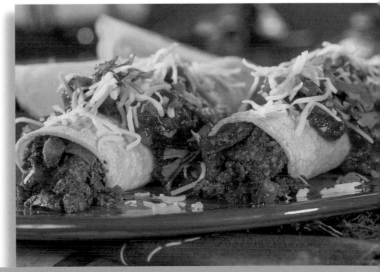

County Fair Steak Sandwiches

Serves 6, 1 sandwich per serving

1	tablespoon olive oil, divided
1	red bell pepper, thinly sliced
1	green bell pepper, thinly sliced
1	onion, cut in half and thinly sliced
1/2	teaspoon garlic powder
8	ounces sliced mushrooms
1	pound beef sirloin, well trimmed and thinly sliced
1/8	teaspoon salt (optional)
1/4	teaspoon black pepper
1	(1-pound) French bread loaf, cut in half lengthwise and insides scooped out
3/4	cup (3 ounces) reduced-fat shredded sharp Cheddar cheese

1 In a large skillet over medium-high heat, heat 2 teaspoons oil. Add bell peppers, onion, and garlic powder. Cook 6 to 8 minutes, or until tender. Stir in mushrooms and cook 3 to 5 minutes, or until tender. Transfer to a plate and cover to keep warm.

2 In the same skillet, over medium-high heat, heat remaining oil. Add beef slices; sprinkle with salt, if desired, and pepper. Cook 4 to 6 minutes, or just until beef is slightly pink in center. Remove from heat and set aside.

3 Meanwhile, preheat broiler. Place bread halves, cut side up, on a baking sheet. Place bread 5 to 6 inches from heat for 1 to 2 minutes, or until toasted.

4 Set aside top of loaf. Spoon vegetable mixture into bottom half of loaf. Top with steak and sprinkle with cheese.

5 Broil 1 to 2 minutes, or until cheese is melted. Place top of loaf over filling, cut into 6 equal pieces, and serve.

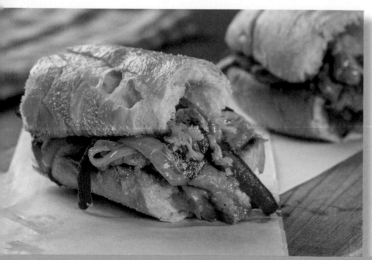

Choices/Exchanges, 2 starch, 1 vegetable, 3 lean protein

Calories 330, Calories From Fat 70, **Total Fat** 8.0g, Saturated Fat 2.5g, Trans Fat 0.0g, **Cholesterol** 30mg, **Sodium** 480mg, **Potassium** 580mg, **Total Carbohydrates** 36g, Fiber 3g, Sugar 3g, **Protein** 26g, **Phosphorus** 330mg

Cheesy Baked Pork Chops

Serves 4, 1 chop per serving

2/3	cup finely crushed reduced-sodium cheese crackers
2	tablespoons sesame seeds
1	tablespoon chopped fresh parsley
1/4	teaspoon salt
1/4	teaspoon black pepper
1/4	teaspoon cayenne pepper
1	egg
4	(4-ounce) well-trimmed boneless pork chops
	Cooking spray

1 Preheat oven to 375°F. Coat a rimmed baking sheet with cooking spray.

2 In a shallow bowl, combine cracker crumbs, sesame seeds, parsley, salt, black pepper, and cayenne pepper; mix well. Beat egg in another bowl.

3 Dip each pork chop into egg, then the seasoned crumbs, coating well. Place chops on prepared baking sheet. Spray chops lightly on both sides with cooking spray.

4 Bake 20 to 25 minutes, or until internal temperature is 145°F and pork is slightly pink, turning halfway through cooking.

Test Kitchen. Mr. Food Hints & Tips

Just in case you were wondering, we spray the breaded pork chops with cooking spray so the coating crisps up like frying does, without all the added calories and fat. Plus it's a lot easier to "oven fry" than pan fry.

Choices/Exchanges, 1/2 starch, 4 lean protein

Calories 240, Calories From Fat 80, **Total Fat** 9.0g, Saturated Fat 2.5g, Trans Fat 0.0g, **Cholesterol** 115mg, **Sodium** 430mg, **Potassium** 600mg, **Total Carbohydrates** 8g, Fiber <1g, Sugar 0g, **Protein** 29g, **Phosphorus** 390mg

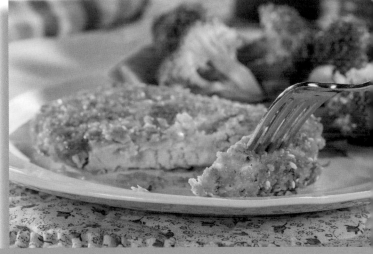

Veggie-Stuffed Pork Chops

Serves 4, 1 chop per serving

1	tablespoon olive oil
1	small zucchini, shredded
1	medium carrot, shredded
1	small red bell pepper, finely diced
1	small onion, finely diced
2	cloves garlic, minced
1	teaspoon Italian seasoning
4	(4-ounce) well-trimmed boneless pork chops
1	tablespoon garlic powder
1	tablespoon paprika
1/2	teaspoon salt (optional)
1/2	teaspoon black pepper

1 Preheat oven to 350°F. Lightly coat a 9 × 13-inch baking dish with cooking spray.

2 In a skillet over medium-high heat, heat oil. Add zucchini, carrot, bell pepper, onion, garlic, and Italian seasoning, and sauté 5 to 7 minutes, or until softened; set aside.

3 On a flat surface, butterfly each pork chop, cutting horizontally 3/4 of the way through. (You can always ask your butcher to butterfly them for you.) Open each like a book. Place an equal amount of the vegetable mixture on half of each chop. Fold tops over, and place chops into prepared baking dish.

4 In a small bowl, mix the remaining ingredients and rub mixture over chops.

5 Bake 25 to 30 minutes, or until internal temperature of the pork is 145°F and pork is just slightly pink.

Did You Know?

Cooking pork to 145°F will leave some pink in the meat. A few years ago, the USDA revised their guidelines, and this cooking method is not only safe, it also keeps our pork really juicy.

Choices/Exchanges, 2 vegetable, 3 lean protein

Calories 200, Calories From Fat 50, **Total Fat** 6.0g, Saturated Fat 1.5g, Trans Fat 0.0g, **Cholesterol** 60mg, **Sodium** 220mg, **Potassium** 800mg, **Total Carbohydrates** 8g, Fiber 2g, Sugar 3g, **Protein** 27g, **Phosphorus** 355mg

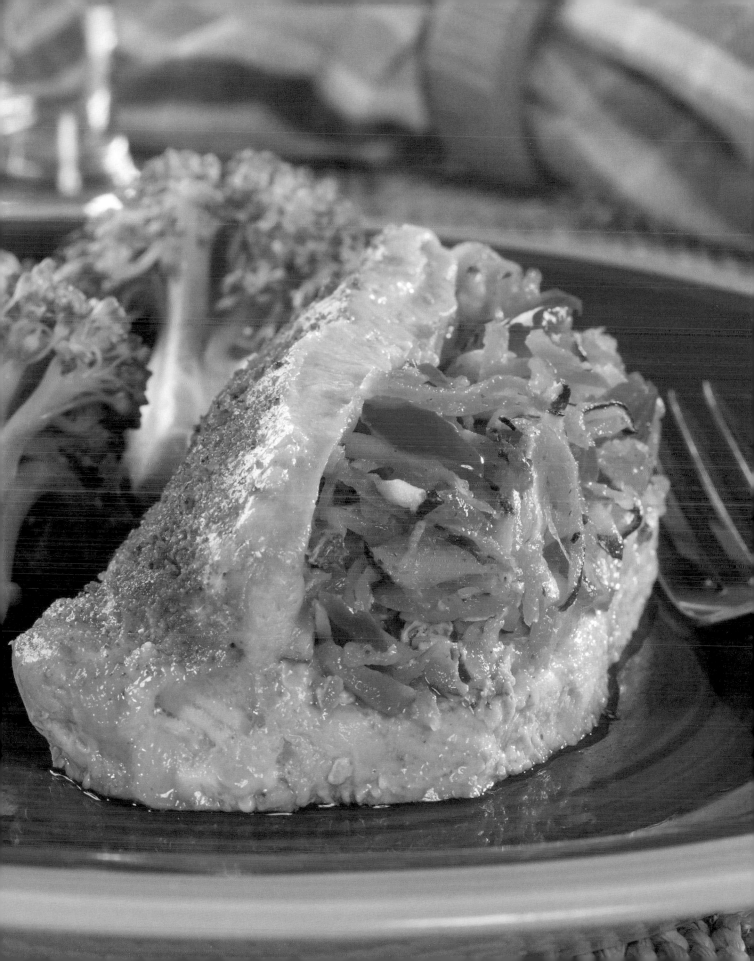

Apple Orchard Roast Pork

Serves 4, 1/4 recipe per serving

1	(1-pound) well-trimmed pork tenderloin
1/2	teaspoon salt
1/8	teaspoon cayenne pepper
2	Granny Smith apples, cored and chopped
1/4	cup water
1/2	teaspoon cinnamon
1/4	cup sugar-free maple syrup

1 Preheat oven to 350°F. Coat a 9 × 13-inch baking dish with cooking spray.

2 Place tenderloin in baking dish and season with salt and cayenne pepper.

3 Coat a skillet with cooking spray. Cook apples over high heat 4 to 5 minutes, or until lightly brown, stirring occasionally. Add water and cinnamon; cover and simmer 8 to 10 minutes, or until apples are tender. Remove cover, increase heat, and stir until liquid evaporates.

4 Stir in syrup until apples are evenly coated. Pour over tenderloin and bake 25 to 30 minutes, or until internal temperature is 145°F and pork is slightly pink, basting occasionally with pan juices. Slice and serve with apples and glaze.

Serving Suggestion

To round out this autumn-inspired recipe, serve pork with mashed sweet potatoes and steamed green beans. Talk about delicious!

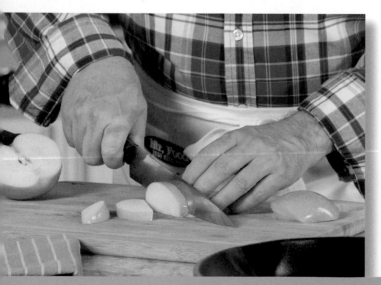

Choices/Exchanges, 1 fruit, 3 lean protein

Calories 200, Calories From Fat 35, **Total Fat** 4.0g, Saturated Fat 1.5g, Trans Fat 0.0g, **Cholesterol** 75mg, **Sodium** 380mg, **Potassium** 540mg, **Total Carbohydrates** 19g, Fiber 3g, Sugar 12g, **Protein** 24g, **Phosphorus** 270mg

Onion-Smothered Pork Chops

Serves 4, 1 chop per serving

2	tablespoons light, trans-fat-free margarine
2	onions, thinly sliced
4	(4-ounce) well-trimmed boneless pork chops
2	teaspoons lemon pepper seasoning
1	tablespoon canola oil
1/2	cup balsamic vinegar
1/3	cup reduced-sodium chicken broth
2	tablespoons light brown sugar

1. In a skillet over medium heat, melt margarine; add onions. Cook, stirring occasionally, about 10 minutes, or until onions are soft and caramelized. Transfer to a bowl.

2. Sprinkle chops with lemon pepper. In the same skillet, over medium-high heat, heat oil. Add chops and cook 3 minutes on each side, or until barely pink in center. Transfer to a plate and cover to keep warm.

3. In the same skillet, combine vinegar, broth, and brown sugar, stirring to loosen any bits from pan. Cook over medium-high heat 4 minutes, or until mixture is reduced to a thin sauce. Add in onions, stirring until heated through.

4. Serve chops topped with onions and sauce.

Good for You!

Most smothered pork chop recipes call for a fairly thick gravy as the "blanket" that smothers the pork. Although ours is a thinner version, you're not going to be lacking in any flavor. We promise!

Choices/Exchanges, 1/2 carbohydrate, 1 vegetable, 3 lean protein, 1 fat

Calories 240, Calories From Fat 70, **Total Fat** 8.0g, Saturated Fat 1.5g, Trans Fat 0.0g, **Cholesterol** 60mg, **Sodium** 300mg, **Potassium** 670mg, **Total Carbohydrates** 13g, Fiber <1g, Sugar 9g, **Protein** 26g, **Phosphorus** 340mg

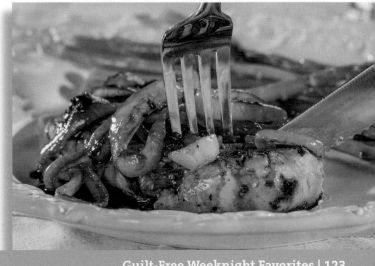

Little Italy Pork Marsala

Serves 6, 1 cup per serving

1/4	cup all-purpose flour
1/2	teaspoon salt, divided
1	teaspoon black pepper, divided
1-1/2	pounds well-trimmed pork loin, cut into 1/4-inch slices
2	tablespoons canola oil, divided
1/2	pound mushrooms, sliced
1	medium onion, chopped
2	cloves garlic, minced
1	small tomato, chopped
1/2	cup reduced-sodium chicken broth
1/4	cup Marsala wine

1. In a shallow dish, combine flour, 1/4 teaspoon salt, and 1/2 teaspoon pepper; mix well. Dredge pork in seasoned flour.

2. In a large skillet over medium heat, heat 1 tablespoon oil. Sauté pork in batches 1 to 2 minutes per side, or until just pink, adding remaining oil as needed. Remove pork from skillet to a plate and set aside.

3. Add mushrooms, onion, and garlic to skillet; sauté 6 to 8 minutes, or until onion is tender, stirring occasionally.

4. Add tomato, broth, wine, remaining salt, and remaining pepper. Bring to a boil and cook 3 to 4 minutes, or until sauce thickens a bit.

5. Return pork to skillet; cook 2 minutes, or until heated through. Serve topped with sauce.

Good for You!

Did you know that well-trimmed pork loin is nutritionally similar to boneless, skinless chicken breast? That's good news, as it gives us more options come dinnertime.

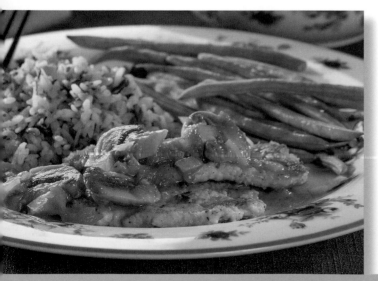

Choices/Exchanges 1/2 carbohydrate, 4 lean protein, 1 fat

Calories 250, Calories From Fat 100, **Total Fat** 11.0g, Saturated Fat 2.5g, Trans Fat 0.0g, **Cholesterol** 65mg, **Sodium** 260mg, **Potassium** 660mg, **Total Carbohydrates** 9g, Fiber 1g, Sugar 2g, **Protein** 27g, **Phosphorus** 295mg

Seafood, Pasta & More

5-Star Salmon Oscar

Serves 4, 1 fillet with topping per serving

1   (1.25-ounce) packet hollandaise sauce mix
1/4   cup light, trans-fat-free margarine, melted
1   cup fat-free milk
1/4   cup all-purpose flour
1/4   teaspoon salt
1/8   teaspoon black pepper
4   (3-ounce) salmon fillets
3   tablespoons canola oil
4   ounces crabmeat, flaked
1/4   pound fresh asparagus, trimmed and cut in half

1 Preheat oven to 350°F. Coat a 9 × 13-inch baking dish with cooking spray.

2 In a small saucepan over high heat, combine sauce mix, margarine, and milk. Bring to a boil, reduce heat to low, and simmer until thickened, about 1 minute; set aside.

3 In a shallow dish, combine flour, salt, and pepper; coat fillets with flour mixture.

4 In a large skillet over medium-high heat, heat oil. Add salmon and sauté 2 minutes per side. Place salmon in prepared baking dish, top each piece with flaked crabmeat and asparagus, and pour sauce over top.

5 Bake 10 to 15 minutes, or until fish flakes easily. Serve immediately.

Did You Know?

To prepare something "Oscar" style means to top it with some crabmeat, asparagus, and either hollandaise or béarnaise sauce. Even though this type of dish is often made with chicken or veal, we think we've outdone ourselves by trying it with salmon. Yum!

Choices/Exchanges, 1 carbohydrate, 4 lean protein, 3 fat

Calories 380, Calories From Fat 220, **Total Fat** 24.0g, Saturated Fat 3.5g, Trans Fat 0.0g, **Cholesterol** 75mg, **Sodium** 600mg, **Potassium** 610mg, **Total Carbohydrates** 14g, Fiber <1g, Sugar 4g, **Protein** 27g, **Phosphorus** 375mg

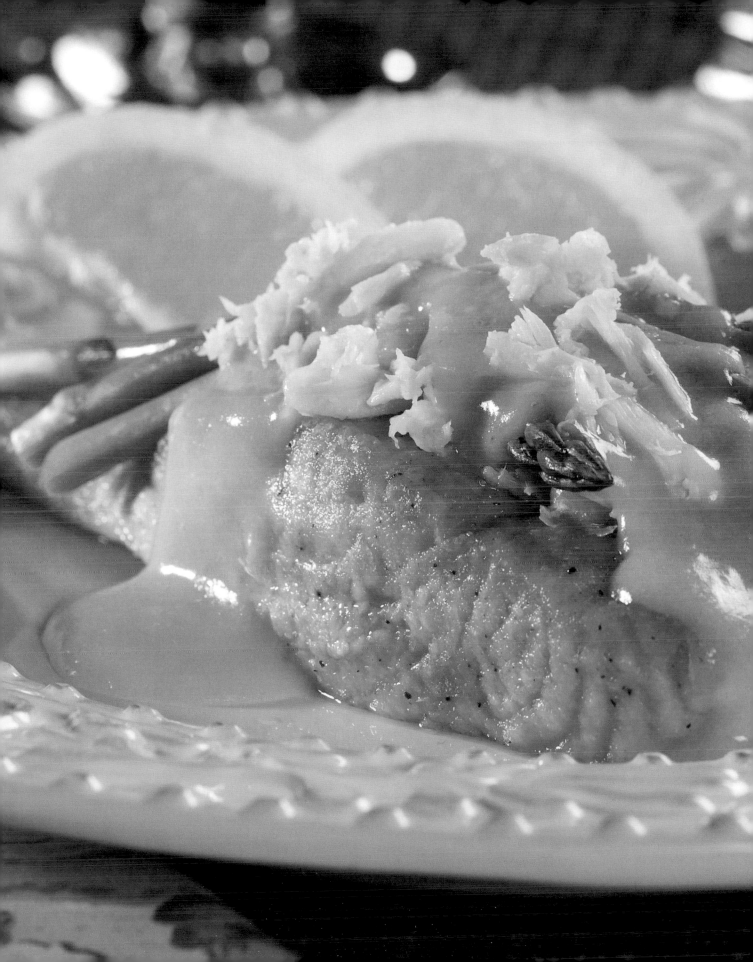

Mississippi Oven-Fried Fish

Serves 6, about 5 ounces fish per serving

1/2	cup liquid egg substitute
1/4	cup fat-free sour cream
1	teaspoon cayenne pepper, divided
1-1/2	teaspoons chopped fresh parsley, divided
1	teaspoon salt, divided
1	cup self-rising cornmeal
2	pounds white-fleshed fish fillets, cut into 1-inch strips
	Cooking spray

1 Preheat oven to 400°F. Coat a baking sheet with cooking spray.

2 In a shallow dish, whisk together liquid egg, sour cream, 1/2 teaspoon cayenne pepper, 1/2 teaspoon parsley, and 1/4 teaspoon salt; beat well. In another shallow dish, combine cornmeal, remaining cayenne pepper, remaining parsley, and remaining salt; mix well.

3 Dip fish in egg mixture, then in cornmeal mixture, coating completely. Place on prepared baking sheet. Lightly coat each fillet with cooking spray.

4 Cook fish 20 to 25 minutes, or until the coating is golden and the fish flakes easily with a fork. Serve immediately.

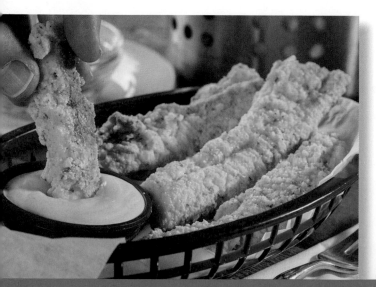

Test Kitchen Hints & Tips (Mr. Food)

Whenever you bread any kind of food, remember to keep one hand wet and the other dry. This way you won't end up with more breading on your fingers than on what you are trying to bread.

Choices/Exchanges, 1/2 carbohydrate, 5 lean protein

Calories 270, Calories From Fat 90, **Total Fat** 10.0g, Saturated Fat 1.5g, Trans Fat 0.0g, **Cholesterol** 90mg, **Sodium** 460mg, **Potassium** 570mg, **Total Carbohydrates** 10g, Fiber <1g, Sugar <1g, **Protein** 32g, **Phosphorus** 510mg

Golden Tilapia Francese

Serves 6, about 4 ounces of fish per serving

1/2	cup all-purpose flour
1	tablespoon chopped fresh parsley
1/2	teaspoon salt, divided
3	eggs
4	tablespoons (1/2 stick) light, trans-fat-free margarine, divided
1-1/2	pounds tilapia fillets
2/3	cup white wine or dry vermouth
4	tablespoons lemon juice

1 In a shallow dish, combine flour, parsley, and 1/4 teaspoon salt; mix well. In another shallow dish, beat eggs.

2 In a large skillet over medium heat, melt 1 tablespoon margarine.

3 Dip fish in flour mixture, then in egg, coating completely.

4 Sauté fish (in batches, if necessary) 3 minutes per side, or until golden, adding more margarine as needed. Remove fish to a paper towel-lined platter. Add any remaining margarine, wine, lemon juice, and remaining salt to skillet; mix well, then return fish to skillet.

5 Cook 2 to 3 minutes, or until sauce begins to thicken. Serve fish immediately with sauce.

Test Kitchen. Mr. Food Hints & Tips

We chose to make this with tilapia since it's a mild white fish, which allows the taste of the sauce to really pop! Plus, since it's nice and thin, it cooks super fast.

Choices/Exchanges, 1/2 carbohydrate, 4 lean protein

Calories 210, Calories From Fat 45, **Total Fat** 5.0g, Saturated Fat 1.0g, Trans Fat 0.0g, **Cholesterol** 155mg, **Sodium** 370mg, **Potassium** 550mg, **Total Carbohydrates** 9g, Fiber 0g, Sugar 0g, **Protein** 25g, **Phosphorus** 295mg

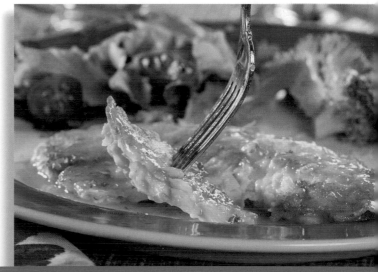

15-Minute Fish Tacos

Serves 6, 1 taco per serving

Coleslaw

2	cups packaged coleslaw
1	orange, peeled, sectioned, and cut into 1/2-inch pieces
1/2	red bell pepper, chopped
1/4	red onion, chopped
3	tablespoons seasoned rice vinegar
2	tablespoons canola oil
1	tablespoon lime juice

Tacos

2	teaspoons chili powder
2	teaspoons cumin
1	teaspoon garlic powder
1/2	teaspoon salt
1-1/2	pounds white-fleshed fish fillets, cut into 1-inch pieces
1	tablespoon chopped cilantro
1	tablespoon lime juice
6	(6-inch) whole-wheat tortillas

1 In a large bowl, combine coleslaw ingredients; mix well. Cover and refrigerate.

2 In another large bowl, combine chili powder, cumin, garlic powder, and salt; mix well. Add the fish pieces and toss until evenly coated.

3 Lightly coat a large skillet with cooking spray. Over medium-high heat, sauté fish 6 to 8 minutes, or until it flakes easily with a fork, stirring occasionally. Sprinkle with cilantro and lime juice.

4 Place an equal amount of fish down the center of each tortilla. Top with coleslaw. Roll up tortillas; secure each with a toothpick. Serve immediately.

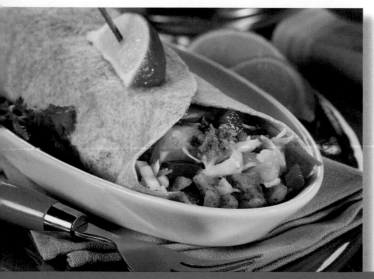

Choices/Exchanges, 1 1/2 carbohydrate, 3 lean protein, 1/2 fat

Calories 250, Calories From Fat 70, **Total Fat** 8.0g, Saturated Fat 2.0g, Trans Fat 0.0g, **Cholesterol** 50mg, **Sodium** 420mg, **Potassium** 460mg, **Total Carbohydrates** 20g, Fiber 5g, Sugar 5g, **Protein** 23g, **Phosphorus** 235mg

Down-Home Tuna Noodle Casserole

Serves 6, 2 cups per serving

1/2   cup panko bread crumbs

3   tablespoons light, trans-fat-free margarine, melted and divided

2   (10.75-ounce cans) low-sodium cream of mushroom soup

1-1/2   cups fat-free milk

12   ounces small shell pasta, cooked and drained

2   (12-ounce) cans chunk tuna in water, drained and flaked

2   cups frozen chopped broccoli, thawed

1/2   teaspoon salt (optional)

1/2   teaspoon black pepper

1. Preheat oven to 350°F. Coat a 2-1/2-quart casserole dish with cooking spray.

2. In a small bowl, mix bread crumbs with 1 tablespoon melted margarine; set aside.

3. In a large bowl, combine soup and milk; mix well. Add cooked pasta, tuna, broccoli, remaining margarine, salt, if desired, and pepper. Pour mixture into prepared casserole dish, then top evenly with bread crumb mixture.

4. Bake 35 to 40 minutes, or until heated through. Serve immediately.

Did You Know?

The Campbell Soup Company is credited with inventing tuna noodle casserole, and the oldest recipe on file is from around 1941. Now it makes perfect sense why the dish is "M'm! M'm! Good!®"

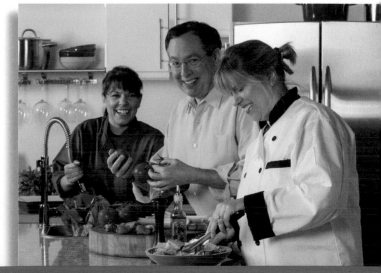

Choices/Exchanges, 3 starch, 1 carbohydrate, 3 lean protein

Calories 440, Calories From Fat 70, **Total Fat** 8.0g, Saturated Fat 2.0g, Trans Fat 0.0g, **Cholesterol** 50mg, **Sodium** 440mg, **Potassium** 560mg, **Total Carbohydrates** 59g, Fiber 4g, Sugar 7g, **Protein** 33g, **Phosphorus** 330mg

Shrimp Salad-Stuffed Tomatoes

Serves 4, 2 tomato halves per serving

3	tablespoons light mayonnaise
1	teaspoon lemon juice
1/4	teaspoon onion powder
1/8	teaspoon black pepper, plus extra for sprinkling
1	cup frozen cooked salad shrimp, thawed
2	teaspoons sliced fresh chives
4	plum tomatoes, halved and scooped out

1 In a medium bowl, combine mayonnaise, lemon juice, onion powder, and 1/8 teaspoon pepper. Stir in shrimp and chives; mix well.

2 Place tomato halves on a serving platter; spoon shrimp mixture evenly into tomato halves. Sprinkle with pepper and serve.

Serving Suggestion

To fancy this up, crisscross a couple of pieces of chive on top of each stuffed tomato. How pretty!

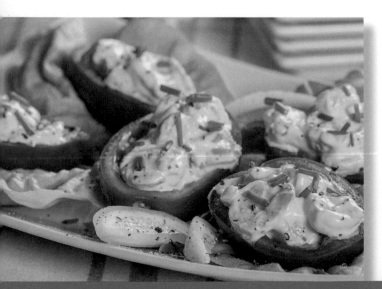

Choices/Exchanges, 1 lean protein, 1/2 fat

Calories 70, Calories From Fat 30, **Total Fat** 3.5g, Saturated Fat 0.5g, Trans Fat 0.0g, **Cholesterol** 45mg, **Sodium** 130mg, **Potassium** 160mg, **Total Carbohydrates** 4g, Fiber <1g, Sugar 2g, **Protein** 7g, **Phosphorus** 19mg

Cheesy Shrimp 'n' Grits

Serves 6, 1-1/4 cups per serving

1-3/4	cups reduced-sodium chicken broth
1-1/2	cups fat-free milk
1	cup grits
1	teaspoon salt (optional)
2	teaspoons olive oil
1	onion, thinly sliced
2	cloves garlic, minced
1	pound fresh or frozen medium shrimp, peeled and deveined (thawed if frozen)
1	tablespoon chopped fresh parsley
1/2	cup reduced-fat shredded Cheddar cheese

1 In a medium saucepan over medium-high heat, combine broth and milk; bring to a boil. Stir in grits and salt, if desired; reduce heat to low, cover, and simmer 15 to 20 minutes, or until grits are thickened, stirring occasionally.

2 Meanwhile, in a large skillet over medium heat, heat oil. Add onion and garlic; cook about 5 minutes, or until onion is tender and lightly browned, stirring occasionally. Remove from skillet and set aside.

3 Add shrimp to hot skillet; cook over medium heat 2 to 4 minutes, or until shrimp are pink, turning occasionally. Stir in onion mixture and parsley.

4 Divide grits evenly among 6 shallow bowls; top with shrimp mixture, sprinkle with cheese, and serve.

Good for You!

One medium shrimp has only 6 calories, hardly any fat or carbs, and more than a gram of good-for-us protein. Maybe that's why shrimp are so welcome in a diabetes-friendly diet.

Choices/Exchanges, 2 starch, 2 lean protein

Calories 260, Calories From Fat 45, **Total Fat** 5.0g, Saturated Fat 1.5g, Trans Fat 0.0g, **Cholesterol** 120mg, **Sodium** 320mg, **Potassium** 410mg, **Total Carbohydrates** 29g, Fiber <1g, Sugar 5g, **Protein** 23g, **Phosphorus** 345mg

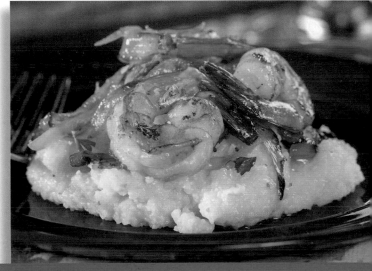

Shrimp & Sausage Boil

Serves 8, 2 cups per serving

8	cups water
1	pound new potatoes (about 2 inches in diameter), halved
1	onion, cut into 6 wedges
2	celery stalks, quartered
1-1/2	tablespoons reduced-sodium seafood seasoning
1/2	teaspoon cayenne pepper
3	ears corn, cut into quarters
8	ounces lean smoked turkey sausage, cut into 3/4-inch slices
1	pound large shrimp, peeled and deveined

1 In a 6- to 8-quart Dutch oven or soup pot over high heat, combine water, potatoes, onion, celery, seafood seasoning, and cayenne pepper; cover and bring to a boil. Cook 8 minutes.

2 Add corn and sausage and cook, covered, 6 more minutes.

3 Add shrimp; reduce heat to simmer. Cook, covered, 2 to 3 more minutes, or until shrimp turn pink and the potatoes are tender, stirring occasionally.

4 Drain liquid from pot, reserving some for dunking (see note); serve immediately.

Serving Suggestion

The broth from this boil is super flavorful. Rather than pouring it down the drain, try serving everyone their own crock of it so they can dunk away! (Just make sure you have lots of napkins!)

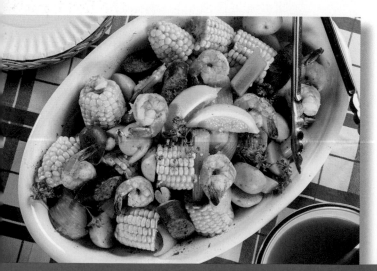

Choices/Exchanges, 1 1/2 starch, 2 lean protein

Calories 190, Calories From Fat 35, **Total Fat** 4.0g, Saturated Fat 1.0g, Trans Fat 0.0g, **Cholesterol** 90mg, **Sodium** 600mg, **Potassium** 480mg, **Total Carbohydrates** 22g, Fiber 3g, Sugar 4g, **Protein** 15g, **Phosphorus** 225mg

Shrimp Waldorf Salad

Serves 4, 1 cup per serving

1	large apple, cored and diced
2	teaspoons lemon juice
1/2	pound large shrimp, peeled and deveined, cooked and diced
3/4	cup seedless red grapes, halved
1/2	cup diced celery
1/4	cup reduced-fat mayonnaise
1/4	teaspoon salt
1/2	teaspoon dill weed

1 In a small bowl, toss diced apple with lemon juice to prevent browning.

2 In a large bowl, combine the remaining ingredients; add apple and toss gently. Serve or refrigerate until ready to serve.

Did You Know?

The first Waldorf salad was created at New York's Waldorf Astoria Hotel in 1896, not by the chef but rather by the maître d'. It was a huge success and has stood the test of time. Let us know on Facebook what you think of our new twist on it.

Choices/Exchanges, 1 fruit, 2 lean protein, 1/2 fat

Calories 160, Calories From Fat 50, **Total Fat** 6.0g, Saturated Fat 1.0g, Trans Fat 0.0g, **Cholesterol** 105mg, **Sodium** 390mg, **Potassium** 260mg, **Total Carbohydrates** 17g, Fiber 2g, Sugar 11g, **Protein** 12g, **Phosphorus** 95mg

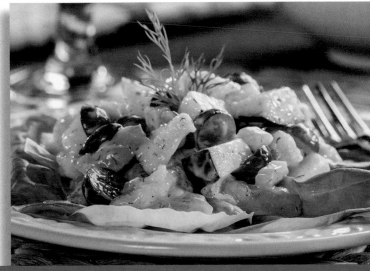

Cauliflower Flatbread

Serves 4, 1 piece per serving

1	large head cauliflower
2	cups (8 ounces) fat-free shredded mozzarella cheese, divided
2	eggs, lightly beaten
2	cloves garlic, minced
1/2	teaspoon onion powder
1/2	teaspoon Italian seasoning
1/8	teaspoon salt (optional)
1/8	teaspoon black pepper
1-1/2	tablespoons pesto sauce

1 Preheat oven to 450°F. Coat a baking sheet with cooking spray.

2 Chop cauliflower into chunks, place in a microwaveable bowl, cover, and microwave 5 minutes, or until soft; let cool.

3 Place cauliflower in a food processor or blender and process until it reaches the consistency of mashed potatoes.

4 In a bowl, combine cauliflower, 1 cup cheese, eggs, garlic, onion powder, Italian seasoning, salt, if desired, and pepper until well mixed. Spread mixture in a 1/2-inch-thick layer on prepared baking sheet. Top with remaining cheese and drizzle with pesto sauce.

5 Bake 20 to 25 minutes, or until golden. Cut into 4 pieces and serve immediately.

Serving Suggestion
Top this amazing "flatbread" with thin slices of grape or cherry tomatoes to add a pop of color and a touch of freshness.

Choices/Exchanges, 1 carbohydrate, 3 lean protein

Calories 210, Calories From Fat 45, **Total Fat** 5.0g, Saturated Fat 1.5g, Trans Fat 0.0g, **Cholesterol** 120mg, **Sodium** 560mg, **Potassium** 760mg, **Total Carbohydrates** 15g, Fiber 6g, Sugar 6g, **Protein** 26g, **Phosphorus** 515mg

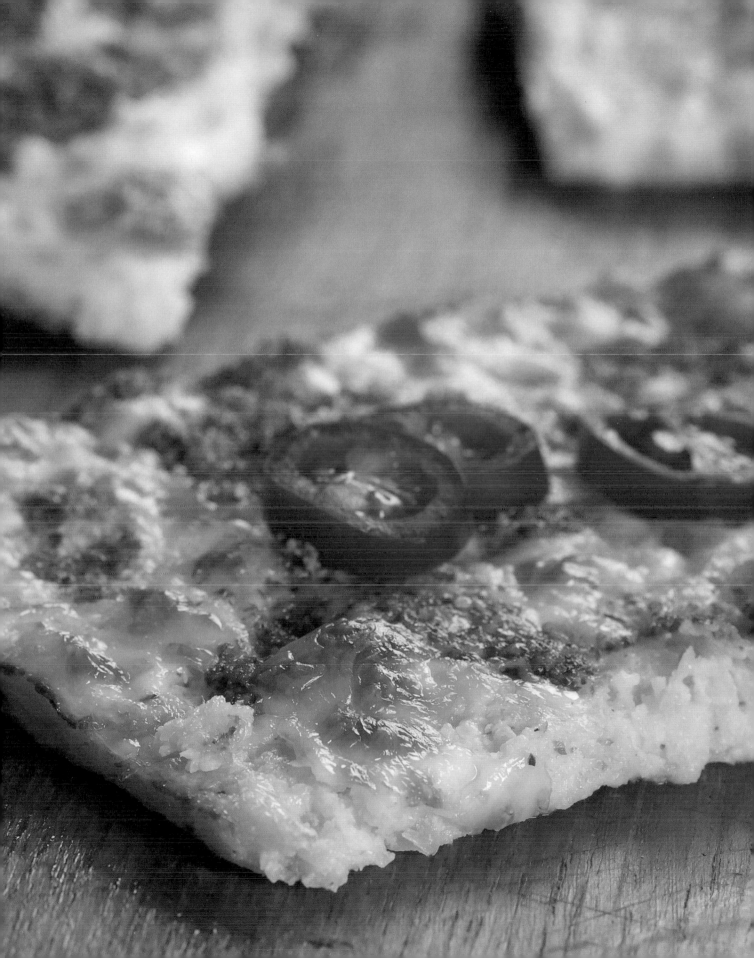

Mama Maria's Chicken Penne

Serves 6, 2 cups per serving

1   cup fat-free milk
1-1/2   tablespoons cornstarch
1   cup reduced-sodium chicken broth
2   ounces reduced-fat cream cheese
1/2   teaspoon garlic powder
1/8   teaspoon salt
1/4   teaspoon black pepper
1/2   cup reduced-fat grated Parmesan cheese
8   ounces penne, cooked and drained
3   cups frozen peas, thawed
8   ounces boneless, skinless chicken breast, cooked and diced

1 In a large saucepan, whisk milk and cornstarch until smooth. Whisk in broth and place over low heat. Add cream cheese, garlic powder, salt, and pepper. Bring to a low simmer, and cook until sauce thickens, about 4 minutes. Whisk in Parmesan cheese and cook 1 to 2 more minutes, or until sauce is smooth.

2 Add penne pasta, peas, and chicken, stirring about 5 minutes, or until heated through.

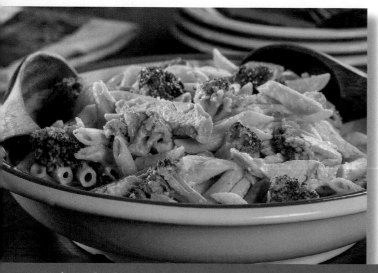

Good for You!

A serving of the typical fettuccine Alfredo has more than 1,500 calories and 40 grams of saturated fat, yet Mama Maria's only has 290 calories and 2.5 grams of saturated fat. We'd say that's quite a significant savings!

Choices/Exchanges, 2 1/2 starch, 2 lean protein

Calories 290, Calories From Fat 45, **Total Fat** 5.0g, Saturated Fat 2.5g, Trans Fat 0.0g, **Cholesterol** 40mg, **Sodium** 280mg, **Potassium** 230mg, **Total Carbohydrates** 37g, Fiber 2g, Sugar 3g, **Protein** 22g, **Phosphorus** 160mg

Miracle Pasta

Serves 6, 2 cups per serving

12	ounces linguine pasta, uncooked, broken in half (see note)
1	(28-ounce) can diced tomatoes
1	onion, thinly sliced
4	cloves garlic, thinly sliced
4-1/2	cups reduced-sodium chicken broth
2	teaspoons dried oregano
1/2	teaspoon crushed red pepper flakes
1/4	teaspoon salt
2	tablespoons olive oil
2	tablespoons chopped fresh basil
1	tablespoon grated Parmesan cheese

1 In a soup pot, place linguine, tomatoes, onion, and garlic. Pour in broth and sprinkle with oregano, crushed red pepper flakes, and salt. Drizzle top with oil and cover.

2 Bring to a boil over medium-high heat, reduce heat to low, and simmer 10 minutes, stirring every 2 to 3 minutes, or until liquid is almost gone. Stir in basil, sprinkle with Parmesan cheese, and serve.

Good for You!

When we tested this for our website, mrfood.com, we tried traditional pasta as well as whole-wheat pasta. Although we prefer the traditional option for taste, the whole-wheat version offers more fiber and less carbs, making it a healthier choice. Try both and see which one you prefer. Maybe try using half and half?

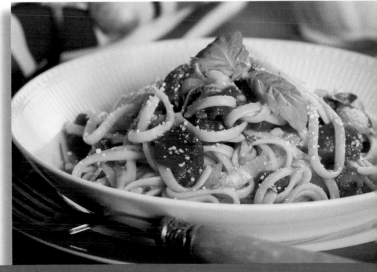

Choices/Exchanges, 2 1/2 starch, 1 vegetable, 1 fat

Calories 290, Calories From Fat 60, **Total Fat** 7.0g, Saturated Fat 1.0g, Trans Fat 0.0g, **Cholesterol** 0g, **Sodium** 340mg, **Potassium** 530mg, **Total Carbohydrates** 46g, Fiber 3g, Sugar 4g, **Protein** 12g, **Phosphorus** 95mg

Veggie White Lasagna

Serves 6, 1 piece per serving

1   (10.75-ounce) can reduced-fat condensed cream of mushroom soup

4   ounces fat-free cream cheese, softened

1   (15-ounce) container low-fat ricotta cheese

1/2 teaspoon garlic powder

2   tablespoons chopped fresh basil

1   large zucchini, thinly sliced

1   (9-ounce) package frozen chopped spinach, thawed and squeezed dry

1   cup shredded carrot

6   uncooked lasagna noodles

1   cup (4 ounces) reduced-fat shredded mozzarella cheese, divided

1 Preheat oven to 350°F. Coat a 9 × 13-inch baking dish with cooking spray.

2 In a large bowl, combine soup, cream cheese, ricotta cheese, garlic powder, and basil; add vegetables and mix well.

3 Spread 1/3 of vegetable mixture in bottom of prepared baking dish. Lay 3 uncooked lasagna noodles onto vegetable mixture. Spread 1/3 more of vegetable mixture over noodles. Sprinkle with 1/2 cup mozzarella cheese. Press remaining lasagna noodles over top and cover with remaining vegetable mixture. Cover tightly with aluminum foil.

4 Bake 1 hour and 20 minutes. Remove foil and sprinkle with remaining mozzarella cheese. Return to oven and bake 5 more minutes, or until cheese is melted. Cut into 6 pieces and serve.

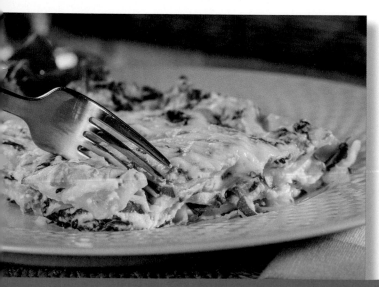

Test Kitchen Mr. Food Hints & Tips

Yes, we do mean uncooked lasagna noodles. The moisture in the veggie mixture will cook the noodles to al dente perfection, plus it helps prevent the lasagna from getting watery from all the veggies. Mangia!

Choices/Exchanges, 2 1/2 carbohydrate, 3 lean protein

Calories 300, Calories From Fat 70, **Total Fat** 8.0g, Saturated Fat 3.0g, Trans Fat 0.0g, **Cholesterol** 25mg, **Sodium** 380mg, **Potassium** 500mg, **Total Carbohydrates** 36g, Fiber 4g, Sugar 8g, **Protein** 22g, **Phosphorus** 275mg

Cowboy Pizza

Serves 8, 1 slice per serving

1	tablespoon canola oil
1	pound boneless, skinless chicken breast halves, cut into 1/2-inch chunks
1	sweet onion, thinly sliced
1	red bell pepper, chopped
1	cup frozen corn, thawed
1/2	teaspoon salt (optional)
1/2	cup barbecue sauce
2	tablespoons canned chopped green chilies, drained
1	(10-ounce) package prebaked whole-wheat pizza crust
3/4	cup (3 ounces) reduced-fat shredded Cheddar cheese
1	tablespoon chopped cilantro

1 Preheat oven to 450°F.

2 In a large skillet over medium heat, heat oil. Add chicken, onion, bell peppers, and corn; sprinkle with salt, if desired, and sauté 5 to 7 minutes, or until chicken is cooked through. Drain excess liquid.

3 Remove from heat and add barbecue sauce and green chilies; mix until well combined.

4 Spoon chicken mixture evenly over pizza crust; sprinkle with cheese.

5 Bake 10 to 12 minutes, or until crust is crisp and cheese is melted. Sprinkle with cilantro, cut into 8 slices, and serve.

Did You Know?

By using a whole-wheat crust instead of a traditional one, you gain fiber, plus it's loaded with lots of essential nutrients. And feel free to substitute sugar-free barbecue sauce, if you'd like. See how easy and delicious a few good-for-you changes can be?

Choices/Exchanges, 1 1/2 carbohydrate, 2 lean protein, 1/2 fat

Calories 230, Calories From Fat 50, **Total Fat** 6.0g, Saturated Fat 2.0g, Trans Fat 0.0g, **Cholesterol** 40mg, **Sodium** 520mg, **Potassium** 290mg, **Total Carbohydrates** 25g, Fiber 4g, Sugar 5g, **Protein** 20g, **Phosphorus** 220mg

Black Bean & Quinoa Patties

Serves 5, 1 patty per serving

1/4   cup quinoa
1/2   cup water
1   (15-ounce) can black beans, rinsed and drained
1/2   cup bread crumbs
1/4   cup diced yellow or red bell pepper
2   tablespoons minced onion
2   cloves garlic, minced
2   teaspoons ground cumin
1/2   teaspoon salt
2   teaspoons hot pepper sauce
1   egg

1 Preheat oven to 350°F. Lightly coat a baking sheet with cooking spray.

2 In a saucepan over high heat, bring quinoa and water to a boil. Reduce heat to medium-low, cover, and simmer 15 to 20 minutes, or until quinoa is tender and water has been absorbed.

3 In a medium bowl, roughly mash the black beans with a fork, leaving some whole beans in a paste-like mixture.

4 In a large bowl, combine quinoa, bread crumbs, bell pepper, onion, garlic, cumin, salt, hot pepper sauce, and egg; add black beans. Using your hands, mix well and form mixture into 5 patties. Place patties on prepared baking sheet.

5 Bake 12 to 15 minutes, or until crunchy on the outside and heated through.

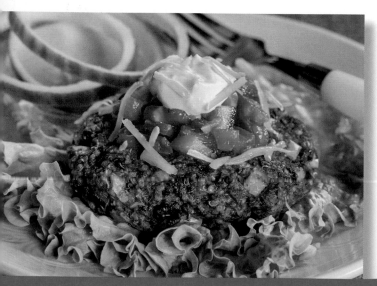

Serving Suggestion

You don't need a bun with these patties. Simply top them with fresh salsa and a small dollop of reduced-fat sour cream, and dig in.

Choices/Exchanges, 1 1/2 starch, 1 lean protein

Calories 170, Calories From Fat 25, **Total Fat** 3.0g, Saturated Fat 0.5g, Trans Fat 0.0g, **Cholesterol** 40mg, **Sodium** 390mg, **Potassium** 150mg, **Total Carbohydrates** 28g, Fiber 6g, Sugar 2g, **Protein** 9g, **Phosphorus** 80mg

Endless Go-Alongs

Zucchini Ribbons

Serves 2, 1/2 recipe per serving

2	zucchini, peeled
1	tablespoon olive oil
2	plum tomatoes, chopped
3	cloves garlic, minced
1/8	teaspoon salt
1/4	teaspoon black pepper

1 Using a vegetable peeler, cut lengthwise ribbons from zucchini, stopping when the seeds are reached. Turn zucchini over and continue "peeling" until all the zucchini is in long ribbons; discard seeds.

2 In a large skillet over medium heat, heat olive oil; add zucchini and cook 3 to 4 minutes, or until softened, stirring occasionally. Add tomatoes, garlic, salt, and pepper and continue cooking 3 to 5 minutes, or until heated through.

Test Kitchen Mr. Food Hints & Tips

Sometimes, rather than having to find different veggies to serve, we can simply change up how we cut or prepare them to get all the variety we need. These Zucchini Ribbons are a perfect example of this.

Choices/Exchanges, 2 vegetable, 1 1/2 fat

Calories 100, Calories From Fat 60, **Total Fat** 7.0g, Saturated Fat 1.0g, Trans Fat 0.0g, **Cholesterol** 0mg, **Sodium** 170mg, **Potassium** 530mg, **Total Carbohydrates** 9g, Fiber 2g, Sugar 4g, **Protein** 2g, **Phosphorus** 75mg

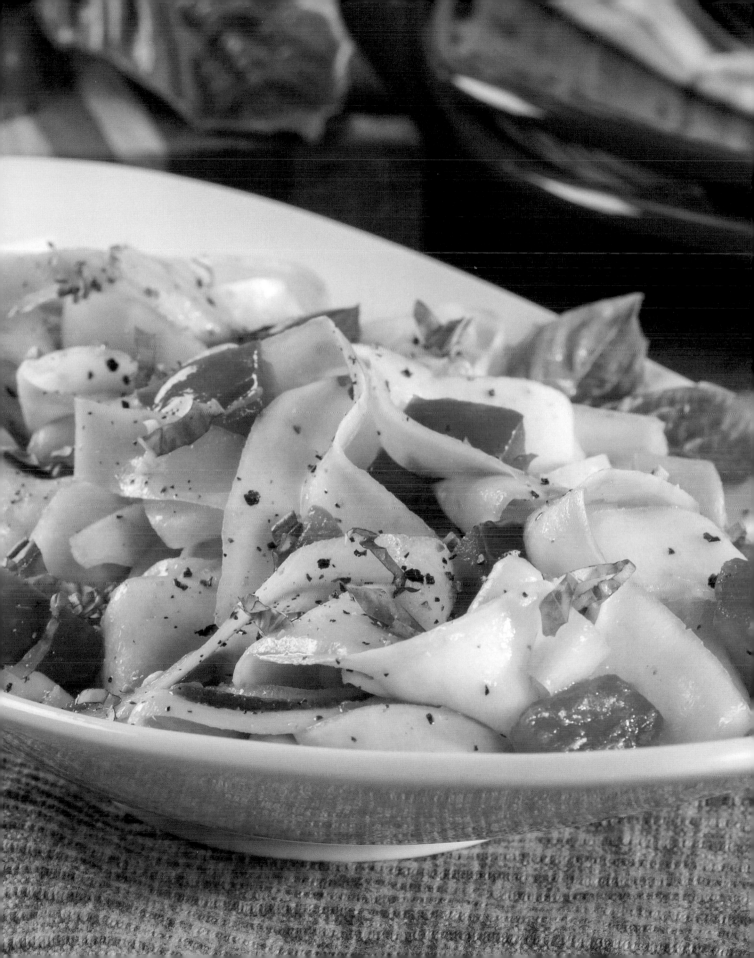

Lemon Roasted Broccoli

Serves 6, about 1 cup per serving

1/4	cup olive oil
1/2	teaspoon kosher salt
1/2	teaspoon black pepper
6	cups broccoli florets
4	garlic cloves, slivered
1	tablespoon lemon juice
1	teaspoon lemon zest
2	tablespoons grated Parmesan cheese

1 Preheat oven to 400°F.

2 In a large bowl, combine oil, salt, and pepper. Add broccoli and garlic and toss until evenly coated. Place on a rimmed baking sheet.

3 Roast 20 to 25 minutes, or until crisp-tender and the tips of some of the florets are browned.

4 Meanwhile, in a small bowl, combine lemon juice and lemon zest. Drizzle over broccoli, sprinkle with Parmesan cheese, and serve.

Did You Know?
Roasting vegetables brings out a nutty sweetness that delivers a ton of flavor without any additional calories or carbs. So feel free to roast away without any guilt.

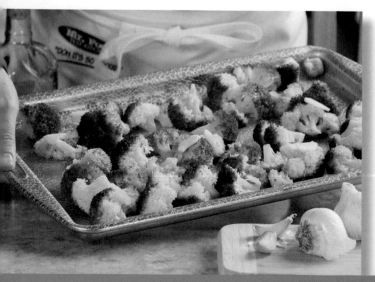

Choices/Exchanges, 1 vegetable, 2 fat

Calories 110, Calories From Fat 90, **Total Fat** 10.0g, Saturated Fat 1.5g, Trans Fat 0.0g, **Cholesterol** 0mg, **Sodium** 200mg, **Potassium** 250mg, **Total Carbohydrates** 5g, Fiber 0g, Sugar 0g, **Protein** 3g, **Phosphorus** 65mg

Pistachio & Cherry Brussels Sprouts

Serves 8, about 3/4 cup per serving

1-1/4	pounds Brussels sprouts
2	tablespoons olive oil, divided
1/2	yellow onion, diced
1/3	cup dried cherries
1/3	cup shelled pistachios, chopped
1/4	teaspoon salt
1/4	teaspoon black pepper

1 Cut each Brussels sprout in half through the stem, then slice thinly; set aside.

2 In a large skillet over medium heat, heat 1 tablespoon oil. Add onion and cook 4 to 5 minutes, or until soft, stirring occasionally. Add remaining oil to skillet; add Brussels sprouts. Cook sprouts 5 to 6 minutes, or until tender and still bright green, stirring occasionally. Stir in cherries, pistachios, salt, and pepper.

3 Transfer to a serving bowl and serve immediately, or keep warm until ready to serve.

Choices/Exchanges, 1/2 fruit, 1 vegetable, 1 fat

Calories 110, Calories From Fat 50, **Total Fat** 6.0g, Saturated Fat 1.0g, Trans Fat 0.0g, **Cholesterol** 0mg, **Sodium** 110mg, **Potassium** 340mg, **Total Carbohydrates** 13g, Fiber 4g, Sugar 2g, **Protein** 4g, **Phosphorus** 75mg

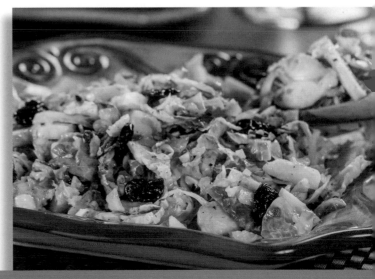

Maple-Glazed Brussels Sprouts

Serves 4, about 1 cup per serving

2	tablespoons canola oil
1/4	teaspoon salt
1/4	teaspoon black pepper
1	pound Brussels sprouts, trimmed and cut in half through the stem
1	tablespoon light, trans-fat-free margarine
2	tablespoons pure maple syrup

1 Preheat oven to 400°F.

2 In a large bowl, combine oil, salt, and pepper. Add Brussels sprouts and toss until evenly coated. Spread in a single layer on a rimmed baking sheet.

3 Bake 20 to 25 minutes, or until tender and the outer leaves begin to crisp. Place in a serving bowl.

4 Meanwhile, in a small skillet over low heat, melt margarine. Stir in maple syrup and cook 4 to 6 minutes, or until mixture is slightly reduced.

5 Pour mixture over Brussels sprouts, toss, and serve immediately.

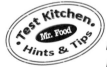

There is a huge difference between pancake syrup and pure maple syrup. Pancake syrup is mostly flavored corn syrup, while maple syrup is the real thing, so a little adds a lot of flavor.

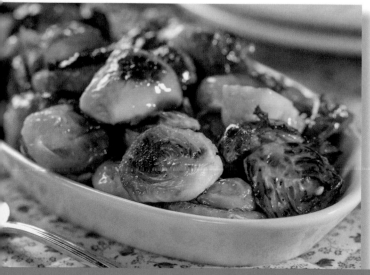

Choices/Exchanges, 1/2 carbohydrate, 2 vegetable, 1 1/2 fat

Calories 140, Calories From Fat 70, **Total Fat** 8.0g, Saturated Fat 0.5g, Trans Fat 0.0g, **Cholesterol** 0mg, **Sodium** 170mg, **Potassium** 460mg, **Total Carbohydrates** 17g, Fiber 4g, Sugar 8g, **Protein** 4g, **Phosphorus** 80mg

Green Bean Casserole Skillet

Serves 6, about 1 cup per serving

2	onions, thinly sliced
2	tablespoons canola oil
1/2	pound mushrooms, sliced
2	cloves garlic, minced
1/2	teaspoon salt
1/4	teaspoon black pepper
2	tablespoons all-purpose flour
1	cup fat-free milk
1	teaspoon onion powder
1	(16-ounce) package frozen cut green beans, thawed

1 In a large skillet over high heat, sauté onions in oil 10 to 15 minutes, or until crispy, stirring occasionally. Remove to a plate.

2 In the same skillet over medium heat, sauté mushrooms, garlic, salt, and pepper 3 to 5 minutes, or until tender. Stir in flour to coat mushrooms. Add milk and cook until mixture thickens. Stir in onion powder and green beans and cook 6 to 8 minutes, or until heated through.

3 Top with crispy onions and serve.

Good for You!

Say goodbye to your old favorite green bean casserole and hello to our newer, lighter, skillet version. This one has less than half the calories, fat, and sodium of the traditional version we all grew up on, yet the taste is still downright comforting.

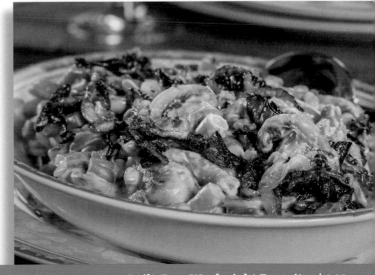

Choices/Exchanges, 1/2 carbohydrate, 2 vegetable, 1 fat

Calories 120, Calories From Fat 45, **Total Fat** 5.0g, Saturated Fat 0.0g, Trans Fat 0.0g, **Cholesterol** 0mg, **Sodium** 220mg, **Potassium** 400mg, **Total Carbohydrates** 16g, Fiber 3g, Sugar 5g, **Protein** 5g, **Phosphorus** 115mg

Tex-Mex Spaghetti Squash

Serves 8, about 3/4 cup per serving

1   spaghetti squash (about 2 pounds)

1   (15-ounce) can reduced-sodium black beans, rinsed and drained

1   (14.5-ounce) can no-salt-added diced tomatoes

1   cup reduced-fat shredded Mexican cheese blend

1   teaspoon cumin

1/2   teaspoon chili powder

1/2   teaspoon salt

1   tablespoon chopped fresh cilantro, plus extra for garnish

1 Pierce squash several times with a fork. Place on a microwaveable plate and microwave on HIGH 15 to 18 minutes, or until tender when pierced with a knife. Remove to a cutting board and allow to cool 15 to 20 minutes.

2 Preheat oven to 350°F. Coat a 2-quart casserole dish with cooking spray.

3 Cut the squash in half lengthwise. Scoop out seeds and discard. Scrape the inside of the squash with a fork, shredding it so it looks like spaghetti, and place in a large bowl. Add black beans, diced tomatoes, cheese, cumin, chili powder, salt, and cilantro; mix well. Spoon into prepared casserole dish.

4 Bake 30 to 35 minutes, or until heated through. Sprinkle with remaining cilantro and serve.

Good for You!

If you're on a low-carb diet, then you will love that spaghetti squash is similar in look and texture to traditional spaghetti, but with only 7 grams of carbs in a cup versus 45 grams in traditional spaghetti.

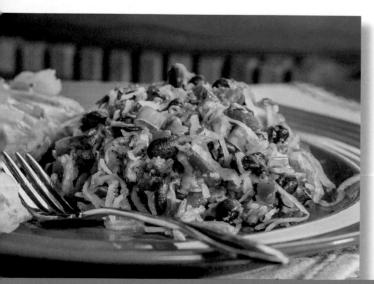

Choices/Exchanges, 1/2 starch, 2 vegetable, 1 fat

Calories 130, Calories From Fat 35, **Total Fat** 4.0g, Saturated Fat 2.0g, Trans Fat 0.0g, **Cholesterol** 10mg, **Sodium** 270mg, **Potassium** 260mg, **Total Carbohydrates** 18g, Fiber 5g, Sugar 5g, **Protein** 8g, **Phosphorus** 30mg

Tomato & Pepper Salad

Serves 7, about 1 cup per serving

1/3	cup olive oil
2	tablespoons red wine vinegar
1	tablespoon sugar
1	teaspoon dried oregano
1	teaspoon garlic powder
1	teaspoon salt
1/2	teaspoon black pepper
4	large beefsteak tomatoes, cut into chunks
1	large yellow or green bell pepper, cut into chunks
2	scallions, sliced
1/4	cup chopped fresh basil

1 In a large bowl, whisk together oil, vinegar, sugar, oregano, garlic powder, salt, and pepper.

2 Add in the remaining ingredients and gently toss until evenly coated. Serve immediately.

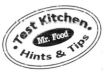

It's best to make this right before serving. That way you don't need to refrigerate the tomatoes, which takes away their fresh taste and can make them mealy.

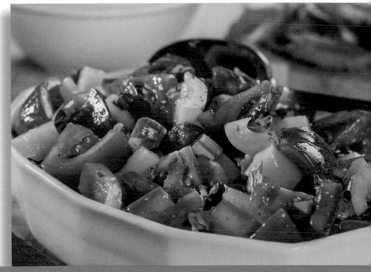

Choices/Exchanges, 2 vegetable, 2 fat

Calories 140, Calories From Fat 90, **Total Fat** 10.0g, Saturated Fat 1.5g, Trans Fat 0.0g, **Cholesterol** 0mg, **Sodium** 340mg, **Potassium** 400mg, **Total Carbohydrates** 13g, Fiber 2g, Sugar 5g, **Protein** 1g, **Phosphorus** 35mg

Grilled Corn on the Cob

Serves 8, 1 ear per serving

8   (6-1/2- to 7-1/2-inch) ears corn, with husks
2   tablespoons olive oil
1   small onion, finely chopped
2   cloves garlic, minced
2   teaspoons chopped fresh parsley
1/4   teaspoon black pepper

1 In a large pot, completely cover ears of corn, in their husks, with cold water; soak 15 minutes.

2 Lightly spray a grill with cooking spray. Preheat to medium heat.

3 In a small bowl, combine oil, onion, garlic, parsley, and pepper.

4 Remove corn from water and shake off excess water. Pull husks back, but do not completely remove them. Remove and discard only the silk. Brush the kernels with oil mixture, then rewrap the corn in the husks.

5 Grill corn 15 to 20 minutes, or until tender, turning frequently. Remove corn from grill and let stand about 5 minutes, or until cool enough to handle but still warm. Discard husks and serve.

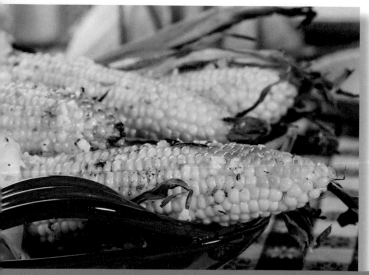

Good for You!
Grilling the corn brings out its natural sugars, plus, since we're using flavored olive oil instead of butter, we cut back significantly on the saturated fats and calories.

Choices/Exchanges, 1 starch, 1 fat

Calories 110, Calories From Fat 40, **Total Fat** 4.5g, Saturated Fat 0.5g, Trans Fat 0.0g, **Cholesterol** 0mg, **Sodium** 15mg, **Potassium** 260mg, **Total Carbohydrates** 18g, Fiber 3g, Sugar 3g, **Protein** 3g, **Phosphorus** 85mg

Garden Zucchini Soufflé

Serves 6, about 3/4 cup per serving

1	tablespoon olive oil
1	medium zucchini, thinly sliced
1/2	cup chopped roasted red peppers
2	teaspoons minced garlic
1	tablespoon chopped fresh basil
1	tablespoon chopped fresh parsley
2	teaspoons chopped fresh sage
2-1/2	cups cubed multi-grain bread
1/3	cup reduced-fat shredded Italian cheese blend, divided
3/4	cup liquid egg substitute
3/4	cup fat-free milk
1/4	teaspoon salt
1/8	teaspoon black pepper

1. Preheat oven to 350°F. Coat a 1-1/2-quart baking dish with cooking spray.

2. In a large skillet over medium-high heat, heat oil; cook zucchini 3 minutes, stirring occasionally. Stir in roasted peppers and garlic; cook about 2 minutes more, or until zucchini is tender, stirring occasionally. Stir in basil, parsley, sage, and bread cubes.

3. Place half the mixture in prepared baking dish. Sprinkle with half the cheese. Repeat layers.

4. In a medium bowl, whisk together liquid egg, milk, salt, and pepper. Pour over bread mixture.

5. Bake 30 to 35 minutes, or until a knife inserted near center comes out clean. Let stand 5 minutes. Serve warm.

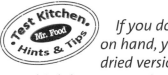

Test Kitchen Mr. Food Hints & Tips

If you don't have fresh herbs on hand, you can substitute the dried versions; just be sure to use one-third the amount since dried herbs are much more potent.

Choices/Exchanges, 1 carbohydrate, 1 lean protein, 1/2 fat

Calories 120, Calories From Fat 45, **Total Fat** 5.0g, Saturated Fat 1.5g, Trans Fat 0.0g, **Cholesterol** <5mg, **Sodium** 290mg, **Potassium** 300mg, **Total Carbohydrates** 11g, Fiber 2g, Sugar 4g, **Protein** 9g, **Phosphorus** 110mg

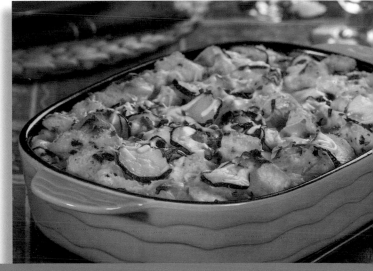

Bacon Mac & Cheese Cups

Serves 12, 1 "cup" per serving

1	tablespoon light, trans-fat-free margarine
3	tablespoons all-purpose flour
2	cups fat-free milk
2	cups (8 ounces) fat-free shredded sharp Cheddar cheese
1	teaspoon dry mustard
1/4	teaspoon black pepper
8	ounces elbow macaroni, cooked and drained
2	tablespoons real bacon pieces

1 Preheat oven to 350°F. Coat a 12-cup muffin tin with cooking spray.

2 In a large saucepan over low heat, melt margarine. Stir in flour; cook 1 minute. Gradually add milk; cook until thickened, stirring constantly. Add cheese, mustard, and pepper, and stir until cheese is melted. Stir in macaroni.

3 Evenly spoon mixture into prepared muffin cups and sprinkle with bacon pieces.

4 Bake 15 to 20 minutes, or until heated through. Let sit 4 to 5 minutes, then remove from muffin cups by running a knife along the edges to loosen. Serve immediately.

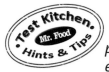

We made these in muffin cups since they're the perfect portion size. This is an easy way to control what you eat, especially when it's this good.

Choices/Exchanges, 1 starch, 1/2 fat free milk

Calories 140, Calories From Fat 15, **Total Fat** 1.5g, Saturated Fat 0.5g, Trans Fat 0.0g, **Cholesterol** <5mg, **Sodium** 320mg, **Potassium** 160mg, **Total Carbohydrates** 20g, Fiber 1g, Sugar 3g, **Protein** 9g, **Phosphorus** 250mg

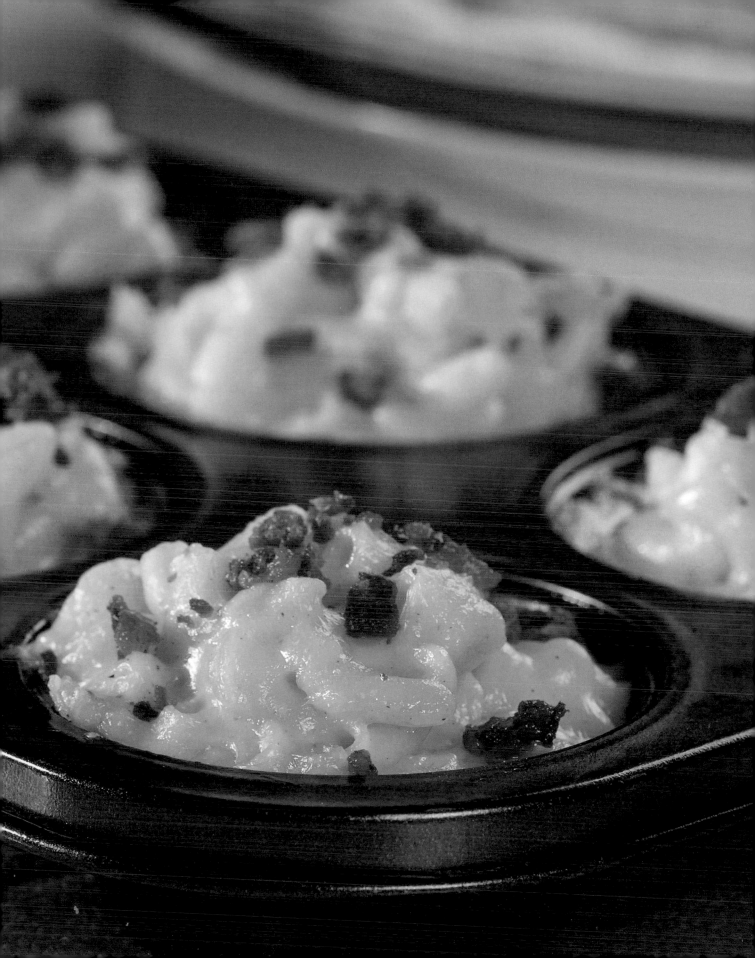

Brown Rice Cakes

Serves 6, 2 cakes per serving

2	cups cooked brown rice, cooled
1/2	cup fat-free milk
2	eggs, beaten
2	scallions, sliced
1	teaspoon minced fresh ginger
2/3	cup whole-wheat flour
2	teaspoons baking powder
1	teaspoon garlic powder
1/8	teaspoon salt
1/8	teaspoon cayenne pepper
1	tablespoon olive oil, or as needed

1 In a large bowl, combine rice, milk, eggs, scallions, and ginger.

2 In a separate bowl, combine flour, baking powder, garlic powder, salt, and cayenne pepper. Stir flour mixture into rice mixture until well combined.

3 On a griddle or in a large skillet, over medium-low heat, heat oil. Scoop 1/8-cup portions of mixture onto griddle. Cook 3 to 4 minutes per side, or until golden brown. Repeat with remaining batter.

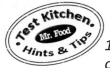

If you prefer to use dried ginger instead of fresh, simply use 1/2 teaspoon. The fresh adds more flavor, yet the dried is more convenient. Decisions, decisions.

Choices/Exchanges, 2 starch, 1/2 fat

Calories 170, Calories From Fat 45, **Total Fat** 5.0g, Saturated Fat 1.0g, Trans Fat 0.0g, **Cholesterol** 70mg, **Sodium** 250mg, **Potassium** 180mg, **Total Carbohydrates** 27g, Fiber 3g, Sugar 1g, **Protein** 6g, **Phosphorus** 185mg

Asian Fried Quinoa

Serves 7, about 3/4 cup per serving

1	cup quinoa, rinsed, if necessary (see note)
1-1/2	cups water
1-1/2	tablespoons reduced-sodium teriyaki sauce
2-1/2	tablespoons lower-sodium soy sauce
3/4	teaspoon sesame oil
1	tablespoon olive oil, divided
1/4	small onion, chopped
2	carrots, chopped
3	scallions, sliced
4	cloves garlic, minced
1	teaspoon minced fresh ginger
2	eggs, lightly beaten
1/2	cup frozen peas, thawed
3	scallions, sliced

1 In a medium saucepan over high heat, bring quinoa and water to a boil; reduce heat to low and simmer 15 to 20 minutes, or until quinoa is soft, translucent, and water is absorbed. Remove from heat and let sit 5 minutes. Fluff with a fork. Place in refrigerator until cooled.

2 In a small bowl, mix teriyaki sauce, soy sauce, and sesame oil; set aside.

3 In a large skillet over high heat, heat 1/2 tablespoon olive oil. Add onion and carrots and cook for 4 minutes. Add remaining olive oil, garlic, ginger, and quinoa. Stir-fry about 2 minutes. Stir in sauce and heat 1 to 2 minutes, or until hot.

4 Make a well in center of quinoa, pour eggs in well, and scramble until cooked through. Add peas and scallions, then toss everything together until warmed through. Serve immediately.

Did You Know?

Some brands of quinoa need to be rinsed before cooking to wash away a bitter coating called saponins. Be sure to read the package to see if the quinoa is prerinsed or if you need to rinse it.

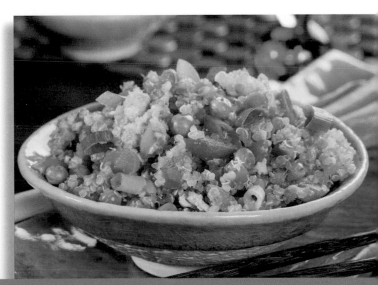

Choices/Exchanges, 1 1/2 starch, 1 fat

Calories 170, Calories From Fat 45, **Total Fat** 5.0g, Saturated Fat 1.0g, Trans Fat 0.0g, **Cholesterol** 60mg, **Sodium** 450mg, **Potassium** 370mg, **Total Carbohydrates** 25g, Fiber 3g, Sugar 2g, **Protein** 7g, **Phosphorus** 180mg

Parmesan Home Fries

Serves 6, about 3/4 cup per serving

3	tablespoons olive oil
2	teaspoons paprika
1/2	teaspoon garlic powder
1/2	teaspoon salt
1/2	teaspoon black pepper
1/4	cup freshly grated Parmesan cheese
4	cups cubed red potatoes
1	onion, thinly sliced

1 Preheat oven to 425°F. Coat a baking sheet with cooking spray.

2 In a large bowl, combine oil, paprika, garlic powder, salt, pepper, and Parmesan cheese. Add potatoes and onion and toss to coat. Place on prepared baking sheet.

3 Bake 20 minutes. Remove from oven, stir potatoes, and bake 15 to 20 more minutes, or until golden and crispy. Serve immediately.

Serving Suggestion

To take these over the top, try sprinkling on some chopped fresh herbs right after they come out of the oven. If that doesn't excite your taste buds, nothing will.

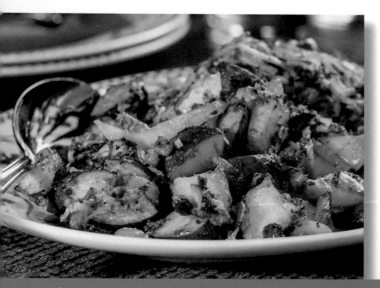

Choices/Exchanges, 1 1/2 starch, 1 fat

Calories 160, Calories From Fat 70, **Total Fat** 8.0g, Saturated Fat 1.5g, Trans Fat 0.0g, **Cholesterol** <5mg, **Sodium** 250mg, **Potassium** 600mg, **Total Carbohydrates** 21g, Fiber 2g, Sugar 1g, **Protein** 4g, **Phosphorus** 35mg

Irish Smashed Potatoes 'n' Kale

Serves 6, about 1 cup per serving

2-1/2	pounds red potatoes, cut into 1-inch chunks
8	cups kale, finely chopped
1/2	stick (1/4 cup) light, trans-fat-free margarine, softened
1	cup reduced-fat sour cream
1/2	teaspoon garlic powder
1/2	teaspoon onion powder
1	teaspoon salt
1	teaspoon black pepper

1 Place potatoes in a large pot with enough water to cover. Place kale over potatoes and bring to a boil over high heat.

2 Reduce heat to medium, cover, and cook 15 to 20 minutes, or until potatoes are fork-tender; drain, then place mixture in a large bowl.

3 Add remaining ingredients; using an electric mixer, beat until desired consistency. Serve hot.

Good for You!

We based this recipe on a traditional Irish dish called Potatoes Colcannon. Our version is "skinnied up" quite a bit from the original version, plus we swapped the traditional cabbage for kale, which is a superfood, so you can feel good about serving this creamy potato dish to your family.

Choices/Exchanges, 2 1/2 starch, 1 vegetable, 1/2 fat

Calories 220, Calories From Fat 25, **Total Fat** 3.0g, Saturated Fat 1.0g, Trans Fat 0.0g, **Cholesterol** <5mg, **Sodium** 440mg, **Potassium** 1450mg, **Total Carbohydrates** 44g, Fiber 5g, Sugar 0g, **Protein** 7g, **Phosphorus** 60mg

Hasselback Creamer Potatoes

Serves 12, 1 potato per serving

12	creamer potatoes (about 3 pounds)
3	tablespoons olive oil
1/2	teaspoon salt
1/2	teaspoon black pepper
1/2	teaspoon garlic powder
1-1/2	cups fat-free shredded Cheddar cheese
2	tablespoons sliced scallions

1 Preheat oven to 400°F.

2 Place 2 wooden spoons parallel to one another and place a potato lengthwise between the handles. Make 6 to 8 crosswise cuts three-quarters of the way through the potato, stopping when the knife hits the spoon handles. Repeat with the remaining potatoes.

3 In a small bowl, combine oil, salt, pepper, and garlic powder; rub mixture evenly over potatoes. Place potatoes on a baking sheet.

4 Bake 40 to 45 minutes, or until tender. Remove from oven and sprinkle tops of potatoes with cheese; bake 2 to 3 more minutes, or until cheese is melted. Sprinkle with scallions and serve.

Did You Know?

Hasselback potatoes are the Swedish version of baked potatoes. These baked potato "fans" were popularized as the namesake dish of the restaurant at the Hasselbacken Hotel in Stockholm, Sweden.

Choices/Exchanges, 1 1/2 starch, 1/2 fat

Calories 130, Calories From Fat 30, **Total Fat** 3.5g, Saturated Fat 0.0g, Trans Fat 0.0g, **Cholesterol** <5mg, **Sodium** 240mg, **Potassium** 480mg, **Total Carbohydrates** 19g, Fiber 3g, Sugar 1g, **Protein** 6g, **Phosphorus** 140mg

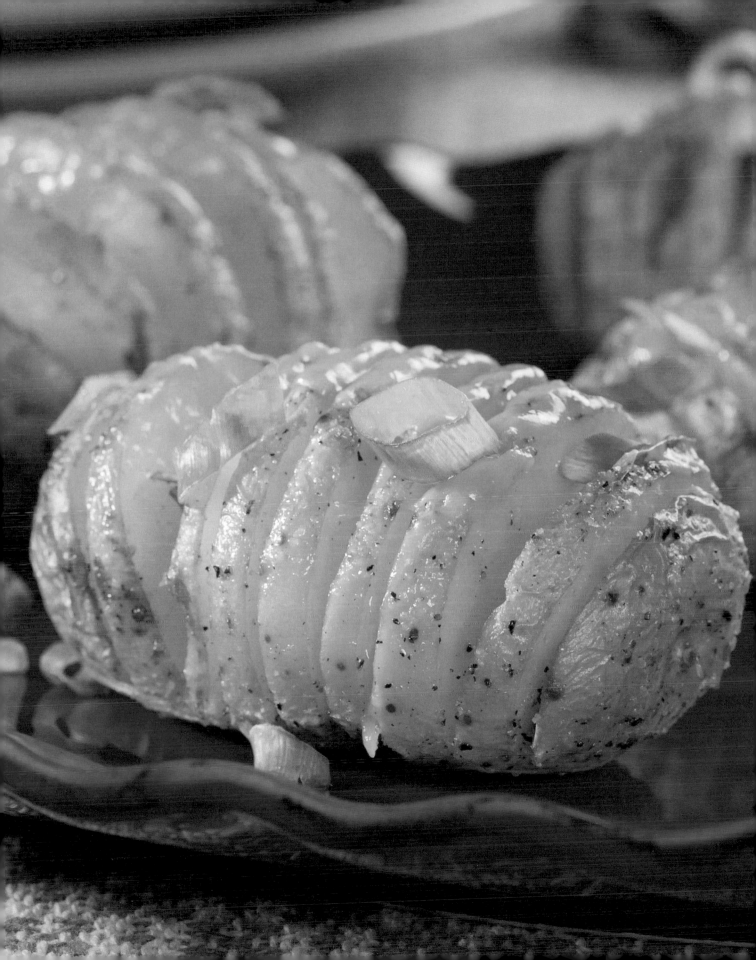

Farm-Style Potato Pie

Serves 8, 1 wedge per serving

1-1/4	pounds russet potatoes, peeled and thinly sliced
3	tablespoons olive oil, divided
1/2	yellow onion, thinly sliced
1/4	teaspoon salt, divided
1/4	teaspoon black pepper, divided
1/2	teaspoon dried rosemary, divided
2	cups baby spinach leaves
3	cups fat-free shredded Cheddar cheese, divided

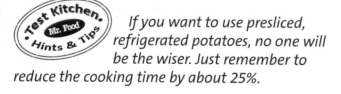

If you want to use presliced, refrigerated potatoes, no one will be the wiser. Just remember to reduce the cooking time by about 25%.

1 Preheat oven to 425°F. Lightly coat a 9-inch deep dish pie plate with cooking spray.

2 Arrange one-third of potato slices in a single layer over bottom of pie plate; brush with 1 tablespoon oil. Place half the onions in a thin layer over potatoes, then season with 1/8 teaspoon salt, 1/8 teaspoon pepper, and 1/4 teaspoon rosemary. Top with half the spinach leaves and 1 cup cheese.

3 Place a second layer of potatoes over cheese, pressing down gently. Lightly brush with 1 tablespoon oil. Continue layering with remaining onions, salt, pepper, rosemary, spinach, and 1 cup cheese.

4 Place a final layer of potatoes on top and gently press down. Lightly brush with remaining oil and top with remaining cheese.

5 Bake 35 to 40 minutes, or until potatoes are browned and tender. Let stand 5 minutes, then cut into 8 wedges and serve.

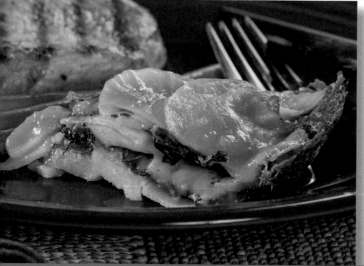

Choices/Exchanges, 1 starch, 2 lean protein

Calories 170, Calories From Fat 45, **Total Fat** 5.0g, Saturated Fat 0.5g, Trans Fat 0.0g, **Cholesterol** 10mg, **Sodium** 500mg, **Potassium** 380mg, **Total Carbohydrates** 17g, Fiber 1g, Sugar <1g, **Protein** 15g, **Phosphorus** 250mg

Southwest Cornbread Muffins

Serves 15, 1 muffin per serving

1	(8.5-ounce) package corn muffin mix
4	ounces (1 cup) reduced-fat shredded Cheddar cheese
1	(4-ounce) can diced green chilies, drained and divided
1/3	cup fat-free milk
1	egg, slightly beaten
1/2	cup black beans, rinsed and drained
1/4	cup chopped sun-dried tomatoes (not packed in oil), rehydrated (see Tip)
2	tablespoons chopped fresh cilantro

1 Preheat oven to 350°F. Coat 15 muffin cups with cooking spray.

2 In a large bowl, combine corn muffin mix, cheese, 1/2 can chilies, milk, and egg; stir just until combined and set aside.

3 In another bowl, combine black beans, remaining chilies, tomatoes, and cilantro. Spoon mixture evenly into muffin cups, then spoon corn muffin mixture over bean mixture, filling muffin cups almost 3/4 full.

4 Bake 15 minutes, or until tops are golden brown and toothpick inserted in center comes out clean. Let muffins stand in cups on wire racks 5 minutes, then run a knife around edges to loosen from sides of pan. Serve warm.

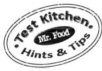

To rehydrate your sun-dried tomatoes, put them in a bowl and cover them with warm water. Let 'em sit for 15 minutes or until tender. It's that easy!

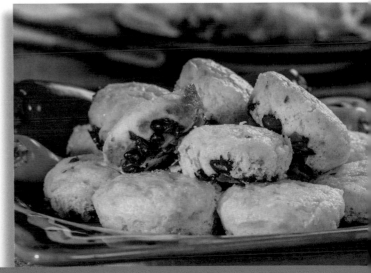

Choices/Exchanges, 1 starch, 1/2 fat

Calories 100, Calories From Fat 30, **Total Fat** 3.5g, Saturated Fat 1.5g, Trans Fat 0.0g, **Cholesterol** 20mg, **Sodium** 360mg, **Potassium** 100mg, **Total Carbohydrates** 14g, Fiber 2g, Sugar 5g, **Protein** 4g, **Phosphorus** 155mg

Crazy Bread Twists

Serves 12, 2 twists per serving

1	(13.8-ounce) package refrigerated pizza dough
1	tablespoon poppy seeds
1	tablespoon sesame seeds, toasted
1	tablespoon flax seeds
1/2	teaspoon kosher salt
1-1/2	tablespoons butter, melted

1 Preheat oven to 425°F. Lightly coat 2 large baking sheets with cooking spray.

2 Unroll pizza dough on lightly floured surface. Using your hands, shape dough into a 12 × 9-inch rectangle.

3 In a small bowl, combine seeds and salt.

4 Brush dough with melted butter, then sprinkle with seed mixture. Use a floured knife or pizza cutter to cut dough crosswise into 1/4- to 1/2-inch-wide strips. Pick up and gently twist each strip, and place on prepared baking sheets.

5 Bake 8 to 10 minutes, or until golden brown. Serve warm.

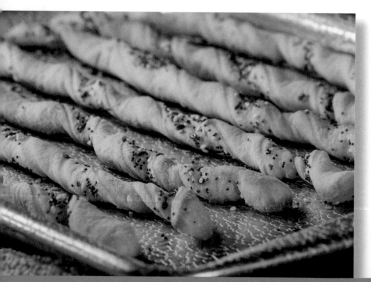

Serving Suggestion

Pair this with our Cowboy Hummus (see page 42) for a perfect snack. The great thing about these is that they are packed with flavor, so they are satisfying. You could say they're "crazy" good.

Choices/Exchanges, 1 starch, 1 fat

Calories 120, Calories From Fat 40, **Total Fat** 4.5g, Saturated Fat 1.0g, Trans Fat 0.0g, **Cholesterol** <5mg, **Sodium** 300mg, **Potassium** 25mg, **Total Carbohydrates** 17g, Fiber <1g, Sugar 0g, **Protein** 4g, **Phosphorus** 25mg

Sweet 'n' Spicy Grilled Pineapple

Serves 8, 1 spear per serving

1	tablespoon sugar
1	teaspoon ground cinnamon
1/8	teaspoon crushed red pepper flakes
1	pineapple, peeled, cored, and cut lengthwise into 8 spears

1 In a large, resealable plastic bag, combine sugar, cinnamon, and red pepper flakes. Add pineapple spears, seal bag, and shake so that mixture coats spears. Place in refrigerator for at least 30 minutes.

2 Preheat grill to medium heat.

3 Place pineapple spears on grill and turn every few minutes, until all sides are grilled.

Did You Know?
Grilling brings out the pineapple's natural sugar, so it's super sweet and juicy without adding a lot of sweetener.

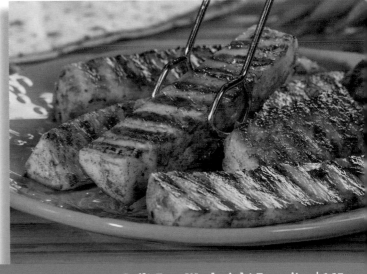

Choices/Exchanges, 1/2 fruit

Calories 35, Calories From Fat 0, **Total Fat** 0.0g, Saturated Fat 0.0g, Trans Fat 0.0g, **Cholesterol** 0mg, **Sodium** 0mg, **Potassium** 70mg, **Total Carbohydrates** 9g, Fiber <1g, Sugar 7g, **Protein** 0g, **Phosphorus** 5mg

Nana's Fruit Cocktail Surprise

Serves 8, about 1/2 cup per serving

1   (8-ounce) container reduced-fat cottage cheese, well drained (see Tip)

1   (4-serving-size) package sugar-free orange gelatin mix

1   (8-ounce) can fruit cocktail in 100% juice, drained

2   cups fat-free frozen whipped topping, thawed

1 In a large bowl, combine cottage cheese, gelatin mix, and fruit cocktail. Gently fold in whipped topping until just combined.

2 Cover and refrigerate at least 1 hour, or until ready to serve.

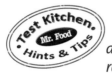

To drain the cottage cheese, place a wire mesh strainer over a medium bowl, spoon cottage cheese into the strainer, and refrigerate for about an hour.

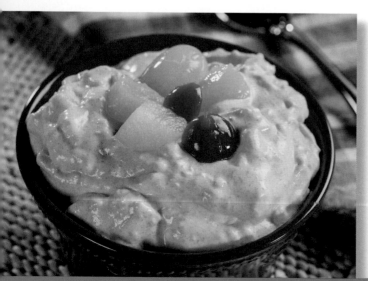

Choices/Exchanges, 1/2 carbohydrate

Calories 40, Calories From Fat 0, **Total Fat** 0.0g, Saturated Fat 0.0g, Trans Fat 0.0g, **Cholesterol** 0mg, **Sodium** 70mg, **Potassium** 50mg, **Total Carbohydrates** 5g, Fiber 0g, Sugar 4g, **Protein** 4g, **Phosphorus** 45mg

Sweets & Treats

Fruit Stand Cheesecake

Serves 16, 1 slice per serving

1-1/4	cups graham cracker crumbs
4	tablespoons light, trans-fat-free margarine, melted
1	tablespoon plus 3/4 cup sugar, divided
3	(8-ounce) packages fat-free cream cheese, softened
1	tablespoon all-purpose flour
1-1/2	teaspoons vanilla extract
3	eggs
1/4	cup reduced-fat milk
1	cup reduced-fat sour cream
	Assorted fresh fruit for topping (we used 1 clementine, 4 strawberries, 1/4 cup blueberries, 8 raspberries, and 1 kiwi)

1 Preheat oven to 350°F.

2 In a medium bowl, mix graham cracker crumbs, margarine, and 1 tablespoon sugar. Press crumb mixture firmly onto bottom and 1 inch up sides of a 9-inch springform pan. Bake 8 minutes; let cool 5 minutes. Reduce oven to 300°F.

3 Meanwhile, in a large bowl, with a mixer on medium speed, beat cream cheese and remaining sugar until creamy. Beat in flour and vanilla until well combined. Beat in eggs, one at a time, beating well after each addition. Beat in milk and sour cream, just until blended. Pour batter into prepared crust.

4 Bake 50 to 55 minutes, or until set but just slightly jiggly. Cool completely in pan on wire rack. Refrigerate overnight.

5 Just before serving, remove side of pan. Place cake on serving platter and top with fruit. Cut into 16 slices and serve.

Choices/Exchanges, 1/2 fat-free milk, 1 carbohydrate, 1/2 fat

Calories 140, Calories From Fat 25, **Total Fat** 3.0g, Saturated Fat 1.0g, Trans Fat 0.0g, **Cholesterol** 45mg, **Sodium** 290mg, **Potassium** 135mg, **Total Carbohydrates** 21g, Fiber <1g, Sugar 14g, **Protein** 8g, **Phosphorus** 220mg

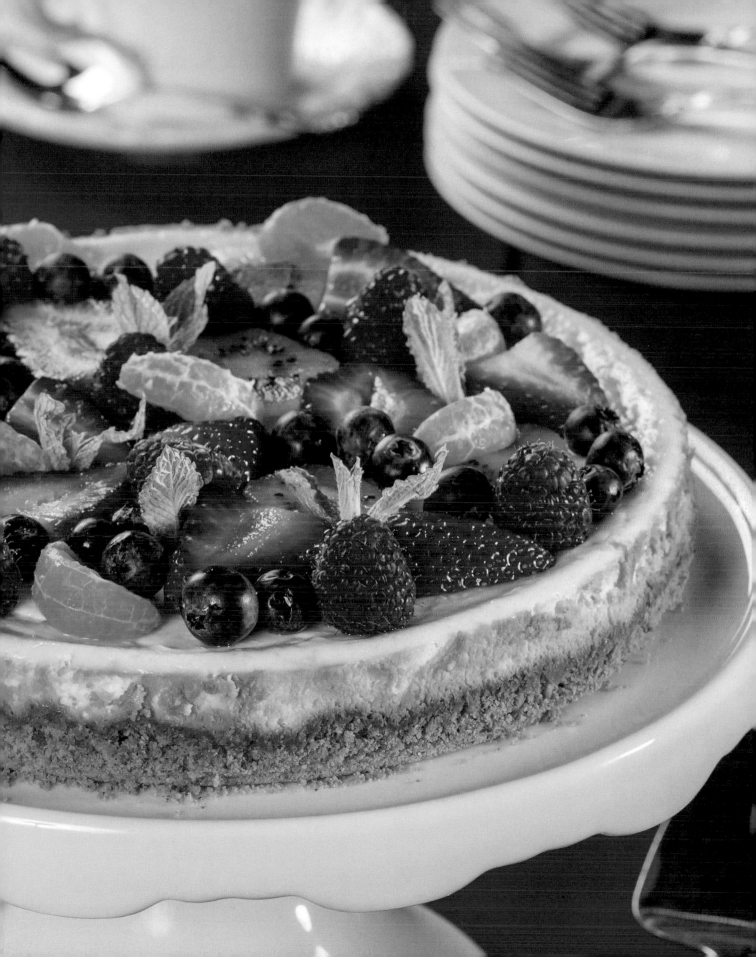

Simple Butternut Squash Cake

Serves 15, 1 piece per serving

1	(16-ounce) box angel food cake mix
3/4	cup frozen mashed butternut squash, thawed
2	teaspoons pumpkin pie spice
1	cup frozen reduced-fat whipped topping, thawed
	Cinnamon for sprinkling

1 Preheat oven to 350°F.

2 In a large bowl, prepare angel food cake according to package directions. Gently fold in squash and pumpkin pie spice. Spread batter into a 9 × 13-inch baking dish.

3 Bake 30 to 35 minutes, or until toothpick inserted in center comes out clean. Remove from oven and let cool.

4 When completely cool, cut into 15 pieces. Dollop each piece with 1 tablespoon whipped topping, sprinkle with cinnamon, and serve.

Did You Know?
Butternut squash not only adds a rich nutty flavor to this cake, it's also the secret to keeping the cake super moist.

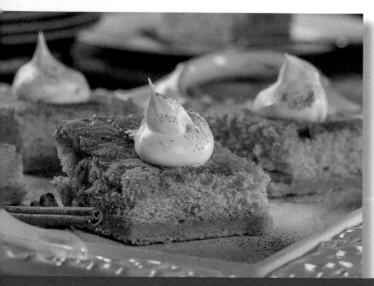

Choices/Exchanges, 2 carbohydrate

Calories 130, Calories From Fat 10, **Total Fat** 1.0g, Saturated Fat 0.5g, Trans Fat 0.0g, **Cholesterol** 0mg, **Sodium** 230mg, **Potassium** 80mg, **Total Carbohydrates** 28g, Fiber 0g, Sugar 15g, **Protein** 3g, **Phosphorus** 110mg

Blue Ribbon Bundt Cake

Serves 16, 1 slice per serving

1-3/4	cups all-purpose flour
1/2	cup granulated Splenda
1/2	cup Splenda Brown Sugar Blend
1-1/2	teaspoons baking powder
1-1/2	teaspoons baking soda
1/2	teaspoon salt
3/4	cup unsweetened cocoa powder
1-1/4	cups low-fat buttermilk
1/4	cup canola oil
1/4	cup liquid egg substitute
2	teaspoons vanilla extract
1	cup strong hot brewed coffee
3/4	cup reduced-fat peanut butter

1 Preheat oven to 350°F. Coat a Bundt pan with cooking spray; set aside.

2 In a large bowl, mix flour, both kinds of Splenda, baking powder, baking soda, salt, and cocoa powder.

3 In a small bowl, combine buttermilk, oil, liquid egg, vanilla, and coffee. Add to flour mixture and with an electric mixer on medium speed, mix about 2 minutes, or until smooth. Pour into prepared pan.

4 Bake 35 minutes, or until a toothpick inserted in center comes out clean. Cool in pan 5 minutes, then invert onto platter. Let cool completely.

5 Place peanut butter in a microwaveable bowl and microwave 10 to 15 seconds, or until peanut butter is warmed. Drizzle over cake, cut into 16 slices, and serve.

Choices/Exchanges, 1 1/2 carbohydrate, 1 1/2 fat

Calories 170, Calories From Fat 80, **Total Fat** 9.0g, Saturated Fat 1.5g, Trans Fat 0.0g, **Cholesterol** 0mg, **Sodium** 330mg, **Potassium** 210mg, **Total Carbohydrates** 19g, Fiber 2g, Sugar 2g, **Protein** 6g, **Phosphorus** 120mg

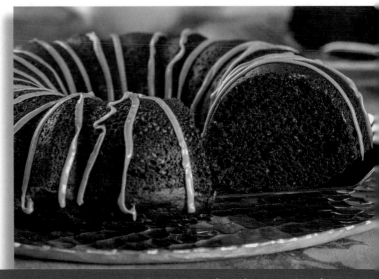

Lime Angel Squares

Serves 15, 1 square per serving

---

2   cups fat-free milk

1   (4-serving-size) package sugar-free instant vanilla pudding mix

1   (4-serving-size) package sugar-free lime gelatin mix

1   (16-ounce) package angel food cake mix

1 Preheat oven to 350°F. Coat a 9 × 13-inch baking dish with cooking spray.

2 In a large bowl, combine milk and pudding mix. Let sit 5 minutes until set; stir in lime gelatin mix. Add dry cake mix and stir until combined. Pour into prepared baking dish.

3 Bake 30 to 35 minutes, or until a toothpick inserted in center comes out clean. Cool completely, and cut into 15 squares.

Serving Suggestion

Sure, these are good to serve just like this, but to take them over the top, try garnishing each square with a slice of lime and a fresh raspberry. Talk about fancy looking!

Choices/Exchanges, 2 carbohydrate

Calories 130, Calories From Fat 0, **Total Fat** 0.0g, Saturated Fat 0.0g, Trans Fat 0.0g, **Cholesterol** 0mg, **Sodium** 320mg, **Potassium** 115mg, **Total Carbohydrates** 29g, Fiber 0g, Sugar 15g, **Protein** 4g, **Phosphorus** 190mg

Éclairs for a Crowd

Serves 20, 1 square per serving

1	cup water
8	tablespoons (1 stick) light, trans-fat-free margarine
1/4	teaspoon salt
1	cup all-purpose flour
4	eggs
12	ounces fat-free cream cheese, softened
4	cups fat-free milk
3	(4-serving-size) packages sugar-free instant vanilla pudding mix
1	(8-ounce) container reduced-fat frozen whipped topping, thawed
1/2	(16-ounce) container chocolate frosting

1 Preheat oven to 400°F. Coat a 10 × 15-inch rimmed baking sheet with cooking spray.

2 In a medium saucepan over medium-high heat, heat water until hot. Reduce heat to low, add margarine and salt, and cook until margarine is melted. Remove saucepan from heat; stir in flour. Add eggs, one at a time, beating well after each addition. Spread mixture evenly onto prepared sheet.

3 Bake 20 to 25 minutes, or until golden brown on the edges; let cool.

4 Meanwhile, in a large bowl, beat cream cheese until smooth. Add milk and pudding mix and beat about 1 minute, or until thick; spread over cake. Refrigerate at least 1 hour, or until set.

5 Spread whipped topping over cake. In a small, microwaveable bowl, microwave chocolate frosting 25 to 35 seconds, or until just pourable. Drizzle chocolate over cake, then refrigerate until ready to serve. Cut into 20 squares and serve.

Test Kitchen • Mr. Food • Hints & Tips

The easiest way to fancy this up is to place the warmed frosting in a resealable plastic bag, snip off one corner, and drizzle the frosting over the cake, as shown in the picture.

Choices/Exchanges, 1 1/2 carbohydrate, 1 fat

Calories 170, Calories From Fat 45, **Total Fat** 5.0g, Saturated Fat 1.5g, Trans Fat 0.0g, **Cholesterol** 40mg, **Sodium** 420mg, **Potassium** 180mg, **Total Carbohydrates** 24g, Fiber 0g, Sugar 12g, **Protein** 6g, **Phosphorus** 285mg

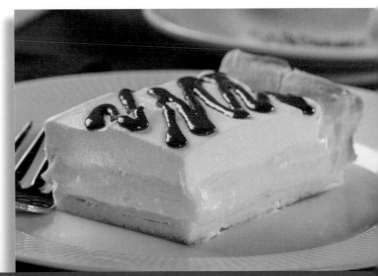

Layers of Heaven

Serves 16, 1 piece per serving

1	(8-ounce) container fat-free frozen whipped topping, thawed, divided
1/2	cup sugar-free hot fudge topping, slightly warmed
1	cup crushed reduced-fat chocolate sandwich cookies (about 8 cookies), divided
11	reduced-fat, no-sugar-added vanilla ice cream sandwiches

1 In a medium bowl, combine half the whipped topping and the hot fudge until well blended. Fold in 1/2 cup crushed cookies.

2 In an 8-inch square baking dish, arrange half the ice cream sandwiches in a single layer, cutting one or two, if necessary, to fit dish. Cover with the whipped topping cookie mixture. Top with remaining ice cream sandwiches to form another single layer. Top with remaining whipped topping. Sprinkle with remaining cookies.

3 Cover loosely with foil and freeze 4 hours, or until ready to serve. Cut into 16 pieces and serve.

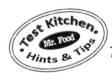

For easier cutting, dip your knife in a glass of hot water. The warm knife will glide right through this like it's butter.

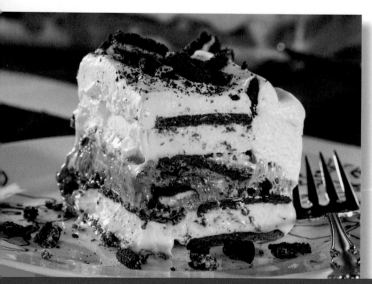

Choices/Exchanges, 2 carbohydrate

Calories 130, Calories From Fat 20, **Total Fat** 2.0g, Saturated Fat 0.5g, Trans Fat 0.0g, **Cholesterol** 0mg, **Sodium** 105mg, **Potassium** 95mg, **Total Carbohydrates** 29g, Fiber 2g, Sugar 6g, **Protein** 3g, **Phosphorus** 0mg

Freckled Blondies

Serves 12, 1 bar per serving

1/3	cup whole-wheat flour
1/3	cup all-purpose flour
1/4	cup packed brown sugar
1/2	teaspoon baking powder
1/4	teaspoon salt
1	egg
1/4	cup canola oil
2	tablespoons honey
1	teaspoon vanilla extract
1/2	cup semisweet chocolate chips

1 Preheat oven to 350°F. Coat an 8-inch square baking dish with cooking spray.

2 In a small bowl, combine the flours, brown sugar, baking powder, and salt.

3 In another small bowl, whisk together the egg, oil, honey, and vanilla. Stir into dry ingredients just until combined. Stir in chocolate chips. (Batter will be thick.) Spread into prepared pan.

4 Bake 17 to 20 minutes, or until a toothpick inserted in center comes out clean. Cool on a wire rack. Cut into 12 bars.

Good for You!

We took the taste and texture of our favorite blondie and tweaked it here and there to lighten it up. What we ended up with are bars that have less than half the calories, fat, and carbs. Now that's a reason to celebrate!

Choices/Exchanges, 1 carbohydrate, 1 1/2 fat

Calories 130, Calories From Fat 60, **Total Fat** 7.0g, Saturated Fat 1.5g, Trans Fat 0.0g, **Cholesterol** 20mg, **Sodium** 80mg, **Potassium** 40mg, **Total Carbohydrates** 17g, Fiber <1g, Sugar 7g, **Protein** 2g, **Phosphorus** 30mg

Fudgy Turtle Cookies

Serves 36, 1 cookie per serving

1	(16-ounce) package sugar-free devil's food cake mix
1/3	cup canola oil
2	eggs
2	(3-ounce) packages (about 12 pieces) sugar-free pecan, caramel, and chocolate candies, coarsely chopped (we tested this with Russell Stover)
1/2	cup sugar-free caramel syrup

1 Preheat oven to 350°F. Coat 2 baking sheets with cooking spray.

2 In a large bowl, combine cake mix, oil, and eggs, and beat with an electric mixer 3 to 4 minutes, or until well blended. With a spoon, stir in chopped candy, then drop by teaspoonfuls 2 inches apart onto prepared baking sheets.

3 Bake 9 to 11 minutes, or until centers of cookies are set. Remove cookies to a wire rack to cool completely. Drizzle with caramel syrup and serve.

Did You Know?
No, silly, these don't have turtles in them. We call 'em turtle cookies after turtle candies (which are pecans laced with caramel and chocolate), which often resemble turtles with the legs sticking out.

Choices/Exchanges, 1/2 carbohydrate, 1/2 fat

Calories 50, Calories From Fat 35, **Total Fat** 4.0g, Saturated Fat 1.0g, Trans Fat 0.0g, **Cholesterol** 10mg, **Sodium** 15mg, **Potassium** 0mg, **Total Carbohydrates** 6g, Fiber 0g, Sugar 0g, **Protein** <1g, **Phosphorus** 5mg

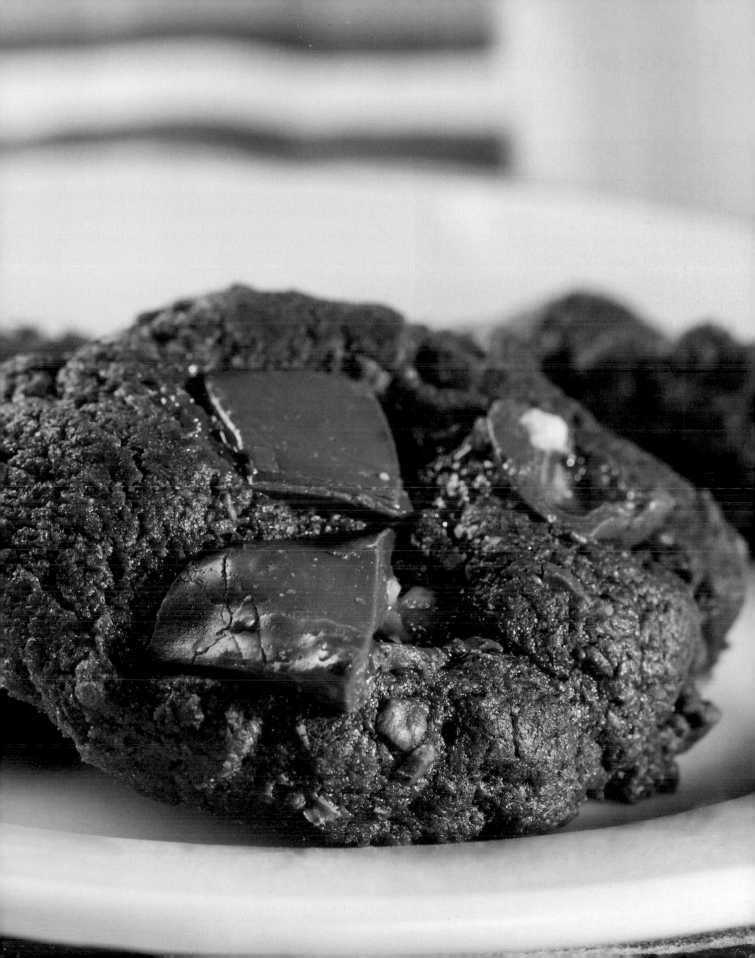

Homestyle Peanut Butter Cookies

Serves 20, 1 cookie per serving

1	cup creamy peanut butter
1-1/4	cups Splenda Sugar Blend, divided
1	large egg
1	teaspoon vanilla extract
2	tablespoons chopped peanuts

1 Preheat oven to 375°F. Coat 2 baking sheets with cooking spray.

2 In a medium bowl, stir together peanut butter, 1 cup Splenda, egg, and vanilla extract.

3 Using your hands, roll mixture into 1-inch balls; place 2 inches apart on prepared baking sheets. Flatten each ball slightly with a drinking glass that has been lightly greased and dipped in remaining Splenda. Sprinkle with chopped peanuts.

4 Bake 8 to 9 minutes, or until edges are set and bottoms are lightly browned. Cool on a wire baking rack.

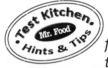

No, we didn't make a mistake, these cookies don't have any flour in them. It's the combo of the peanut butter and the egg that gives them their texture.

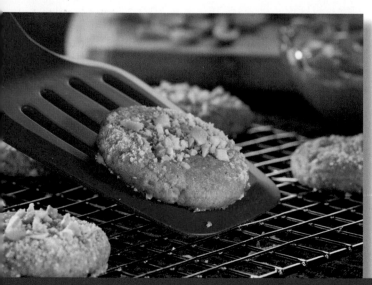

Choices/Exchanges, 1/2 carbohydrate, 1 1/2 fat

Calories 110, Calories From Fat 70, **Total Fat** 8.0g, Saturated Fat 1.5g, Trans Fat 0.0g, **Cholesterol** 10mg, **Sodium** 90mg, **Potassium** 95mg, **Total Carbohydrates** 5g, Fiber <1g, Sugar 3g, **Protein** 4g, **Phosphorus** 60mg

Polka Dot Cookies

Serves 20, 1 cookie per serving

1	cup all-purpose flour
1/4	teaspoon baking soda
4	tablespoons (1/4 cup) light, trans-fat-free margarine
2/3	cup granulated sugar
1/3	cup unsweetened cocoa powder
1/4	cup packed brown sugar
1/8	teaspoon cinnamon
1/4	cup buttermilk
1	teaspoon vanilla extract
1/2	cup white chocolate chips

1 In a small bowl, combine flour and baking soda; set aside.

2 In a saucepan, melt margarine and remove from heat. Stir in granulated sugar, cocoa powder, brown sugar, and cinnamon. Stir in buttermilk and vanilla. Stir in flour mixture just until combined. Stir in white chocolate chips. Cover and refrigerate 1 hour.

3 Meanwhile, preheat oven to 350°F. Lightly coat 2 baking sheets with cooking spray.

4 Shape dough into 1-inch balls and place on prepared baking sheets. Flatten each ball gently.

5 Bake 8 to 10 minutes, or until edges are set. Cool slightly before serving

Test Kitchen. Mr. Food Hints & Tips

Don't have any buttermilk on hand? To make an easy equivalent, place 3/4 teaspoon white vinegar in a measuring cup. Add enough milk to make 1/4 cup total and stir. Let stand for 5 minutes before using. Ta-da ... you now have buttermilk.

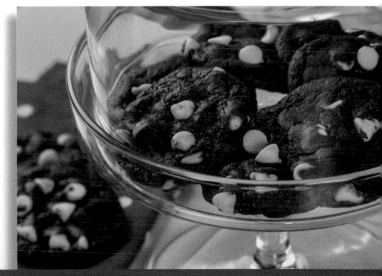

Choices/Exchanges, 1 carbohydrate, 1/2 fat

Calories 90, Calories From Fat 20, **Total Fat** 2.0g, Saturated Fat 1.5g, Trans Fat 0.0g, **Cholesterol** 0mg, **Sodium** 25mg, **Potassium** 45mg, **Total Carbohydrates** 18g, Fiber <1g, Sugar 12g, **Protein** 1g, **Phosphorus** 20mg

Zebra Biscotti

Serves 24, 1 biscotti per serving

1	cup all-purpose flour
1/2	cup sugar
1/3	cup unsweetened cocoa powder
1/2	teaspoon baking soda
1/8	teaspoon salt
2	eggs
1/2	teaspoon vanilla extract
1/2	cup whole almonds
1/2	cup white chocolate chips

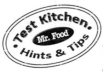

When melting chocolate in the microwave, you want to make sure you don't overheat it. Since microwaves vary in power, we think it's best to only put chocolate in for about 15 seconds at a time.

1 Preheat oven to 350°F. Coat a rimmed baking sheet with cooking spray.

2 In a large bowl, combine flour, sugar, cocoa, baking soda, salt, eggs, and vanilla; mix well with a spoon. Stir in almonds until well blended. (The dough will be thick and sticky.) Divide the dough into 2 equal pieces and shape into 6-inch loaves. Place loaves on prepared baking sheet 2 inches apart.

3 Bake 25 minutes. Reduce temperature to 325°F. Remove from oven and allow to cool 15 minutes.

4 Cut loaves into 1/2-inch slices. Lay the slices cut-side down on the baking sheet, and bake 15 more minutes. Turn biscotti over and bake another 15 minutes, or until very crisp.

5 Meanwhile, in a small, microwaveable bowl, melt chocolate chips in microwave 30 to 60 seconds, or until smooth, stirring every 15 seconds. Spoon chocolate into a resealable plastic bag and snip off a small piece of the corner. Squeeze the bag to drizzle the chocolate over the biscotti. Let sit at room temperature to set. Store in an airtight container.

Choices/Exchanges, 1 carbohydrate, 1/2 fat

Calories 80, Calories From Fat 25, **Total Fat** 3.0g, Saturated Fat 1.0g, Trans Fat 0.0g, **Cholesterol** 20mg, **Sodium** 50mg, **Potassium** 50mg, **Total Carbohydrates** 12g, Fiber <1g, Sugar 7g, **Protein** 2g, **Phosphorus** 35mg

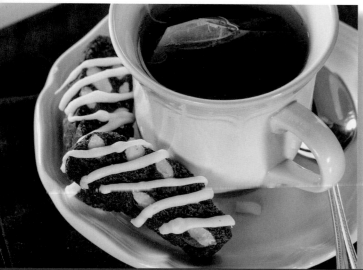

Almond Meringues

Serves 16, 2 meringues per serving

2 egg whites, room temperature
1/2 teaspoon cream of tartar
1/3 cup granulated sugar
1/3 cup confectioners' sugar
1/2 teaspoon almond extract
1/3 cup chopped almonds, divided

1 Preheat oven to 225°F. Line 2 baking sheets with parchment paper.

2 In a bowl, with an electric mixer on medium speed, beat egg whites and cream of tartar until soft peaks form. Add sugar, 1 tablespoon at a time, until stiff peaks form and sugar is dissolved. Fold in confectioners' sugar. Gently fold in almond extract and 1/4 cup chopped almonds. Drop by teaspoonfuls onto prepared baking sheets. Sprinkle with remaining chopped almonds.

3 Bake on bottom oven rack 35 to 40 minutes, or until dry. Turn off oven and leave meringues 45 to 50 minutes, or until completely dry. Store in an airtight container.

Test Kitchen. Mr. Food Hints & Tips

Just in case you were wondering, we add cream of tartar to the egg whites when whipping to increase their volume and help them maintain peaks when being baked. See, ya learn something new every day.

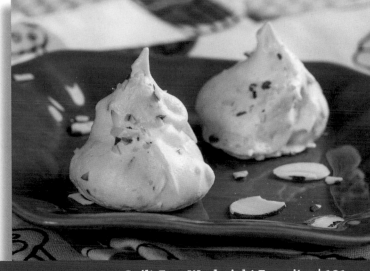

Choices/Exchanges, 1/2 carbohydrate

Calories 35, Calories From Fat 15, **Total Fat** 1.5g, Saturated Fat 0.0g, Trans Fat 0.0g, **Cholesterol** 0mg, **Sodium** 5mg, **Potassium** 45mg, **Total Carbohydrates** 5g, Fiber 0g, Sugar 4g, **Protein** 1g, **Phosphorus** 15g

Tasty Pecan Bites

Serves 28, 1 bite per serving

3/4	cup finely chopped pecans
1/2	cup whole-wheat flour
1/2	cup all-purpose flour
1/2	cup dried cranberries, chopped
1/2	teaspoon cinnamon
1/8	teaspoon salt
1/2	cup confectioners' sugar, plus extra for dusting
1/3	cup light, trans-fat-free margarine
1	egg white
1	teaspoon vanilla extract

1 Preheat oven to 350°F.

2 In a medium bowl, combine pecans, flours, cranberries, cinnamon, and salt.

3 In a large bowl, cream 1/2 cup confectioners' sugar with margarine. Add egg white and beat until light and fluffy. Beat in vanilla. Gradually add flour mixture and beat on low speed until dough forms. Shape dough into 1-inch balls; place 1 inch apart on baking sheets.

4 Bake 10 to 12 minutes, or until lightly browned on bottoms. Transfer to a wire rack to cool completely. Dust with confectioners' sugar and serve, or store in an airtight container.

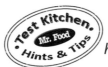

You can add raisins in place of the dried cranberries if you have them on hand ... no problem!

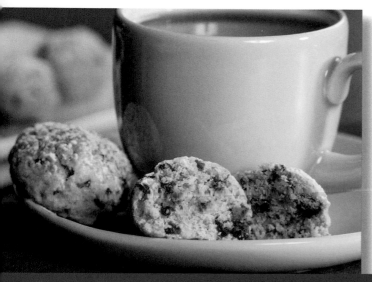

Choices/Exchanges, 1 carbohydrate

Calories 70, Calories From Fat 20, **Total Fat** 2.0g, Saturated Fat 1.0g, Trans Fat 0.0g, **Cholesterol** <5mg, **Sodium** 70mg, **Potassium** 25mg, **Total Carbohydrates** 12g, Fiber 1g, Sugar 0g, **Protein** 1g, **Phosphorus** 30mg

Mini Lemon Meringue Tarts

Serves 15, 1 tart per serving

1/2	cup lemon curd
1	(1.9-ounce) package frozen miniature phyllo tart shells
1	egg white
1/2	teaspoon cream of tartar
1	tablespoon sugar

1 Preheat oven to 375°F.

2 Evenly spoon lemon curd into tart shells.

3 In a bowl, with an electric mixer, beat egg white with cream of tartar until soft peaks form. Add sugar and continue beating until stiff peaks form. Spoon evenly over lemon curd. Place filled tart shells on an ungreased baking sheet.

4 Bake 6 minutes, or until golden brown. Cool on wire rack 5 minutes.

Good for You!
What's great about these, besides the fact that we use a shortcut tart shell which saves us a bunch of time, is knowing that each piece is the perfect portion size.

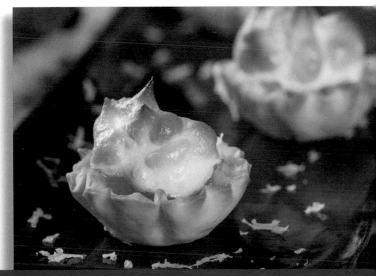

Choices/Exchanges, 1/2 carbohydrate

Calories 45, Calories From Fat 10, **Total Fat** 1.0g, Saturated Fat 0.0g, Trans Fat 0.0g, **Cholesterol** 5mg, **Sodium** 20mg, **Potassium** 20mg, **Total Carbohydrates** 7g, Fiber 0g, Sugar 5g, **Protein** <1g, **Phosphorus** 0mg

Butterscotch Caramel Delights

Serves 12, 1 piece per serving

36	graham cracker squares (each sheet equals 2 squares)
2	(4-serving-size) packages sugar-free instant butterscotch pudding mix
4-1/2	cups fat-free milk, divided
1-1/2	cups reduced-fat frozen whipped topping, thawed, divided
1	(4-serving-size) package sugar-free instant vanilla pudding mix
1	tablespoon sugar-free caramel syrup

1 In a 9 × 13-inch baking dish, evenly arrange 12 graham cracker squares.

2 In a large bowl, whisk together butterscotch pudding mix and 3 cups milk until well combined. Gently fold in 1/2 cup whipped topping.

3 Spread half the pudding evenly over graham crackers. Layer another 12 squares over pudding. Evenly spread remaining pudding over squares. Top with remaining graham crackers.

4 In a bowl, whisk together vanilla pudding mix and remaining milk until well combined. Spread vanilla mixture evenly over top of graham crackers.

5 Cover loosely and refrigerate at least 1 hour. Just before serving, spread remaining whipped topping evenly over top and drizzle with caramel syrup. Keep refrigerated until ready to serve. Cut into 12 pieces and serve.

Did You Know?

Butterscotch and caramel are in the same family. Butterscotch is made from butter and brown sugar, and caramel is made by melting and cooking white sugar. They are both good on their own, but when you put them together, they're amazing.

Choices/Exchanges, 2 carbohydrate, 1/2 fat

Calories 170, Calories From Fat 30, **Total Fat** 3.5g, Saturated Fat 1.5g, Trans Fat 0.0g, **Cholesterol** <5mg, **Sodium** 480mg, **Potassium** 190mg, **Total Carbohydrates** 29g, Fiber <1g, Sugar 13g, **Protein** 5g, **Phosphorus** 290mg

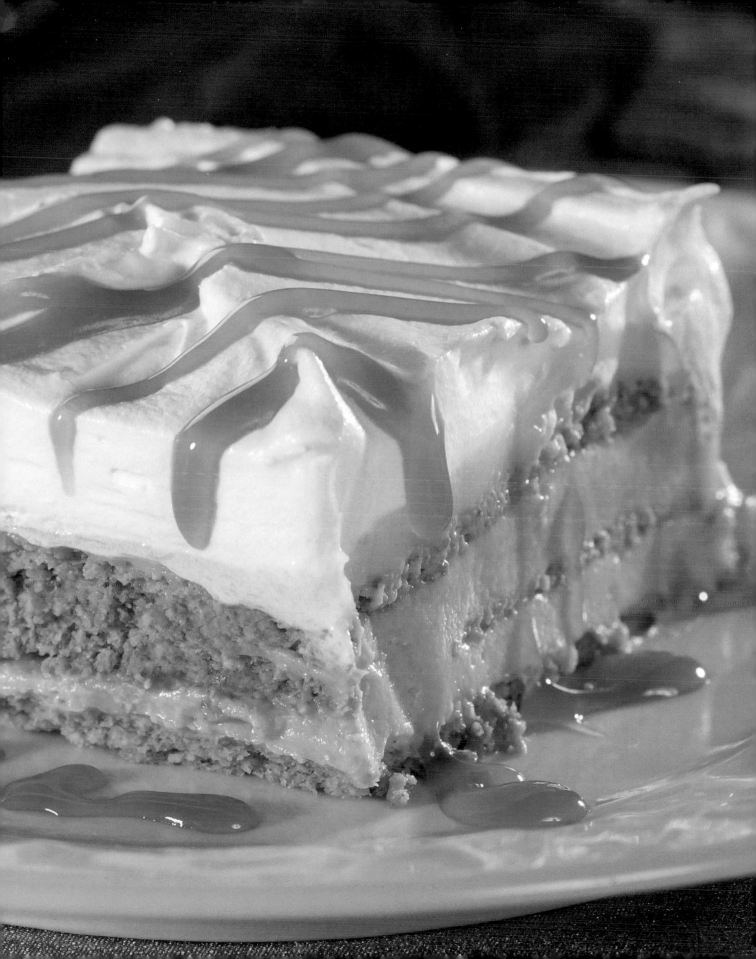

Berry Peachy Crisp

Serves 6, about 1/2 cup per serving

3	cups sliced fresh ripe peaches
2	cups raspberries
1/4	cup granulated Splenda
1	tablespoon all-purpose flour
1/2	cup quick-cooking rolled oats
2	tablespoons brown sugar
3	tablespoons light, trans-fat-free margarine, melted

1 Preheat oven to 375°F. Lightly coat an 8-inch square baking dish with cooking spray.

2 In a large bowl, toss the peaches and berries with Splenda and flour; place in prepared baking dish.

3 In a medium bowl, combine oats, brown sugar, and margarine; sprinkle evenly over fruit mixture.

4 Bake 35 to 40 minutes, or until peaches are tender and topping is golden. Let cool 15 minutes before serving.

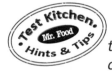

We added a bit of flour to the fruit so that the filling thickens up as it cooks and becomes the perfect, spoonable consistency.

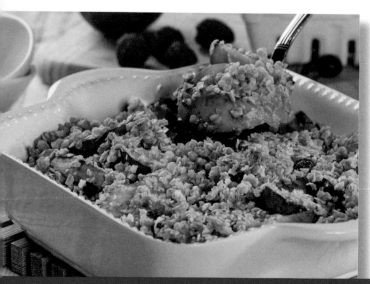

Choices/Exchanges, 2 carbohydrate

Calories 140, Calories From Fat 25, **Total Fat** 3.0g, Saturated Fat 0.0g, Trans Fat 0.0g, **Cholesterol** 0mg, **Sodium** 55mg, **Potassium** 300mg, **Total Carbohydrates** 28g, Fiber 5g, Sugar 13g, **Protein** 4g, **Phosphorus** 100mg

Dutch Apple Crumble

Serves 10, about 3/4 cup per serving

1/2	cup oats
1/4	cup whole-wheat flour
1/4	cup brown sugar
1	teaspoon cinnamon, divided
4	tablespoons (1/4 cup) light, trans-fat-free margarine
1-3/4	cups light apple juice
1/8	teaspoon ground cloves
2	tablespoons cornstarch
6	baking apples, peeled, cored, and sliced (such as Fuji or Granny Smith)

1 To make crumb topping, in a medium bowl, combine oats, flour, brown sugar, 1/4 teaspoon cinnamon, and margarine until mixture is crumbly; set aside.

2 Preheat oven to 400°F. Coat a 9-inch deep dish pie plate with cooking spray; set aside.

3 To make the filling, in a small saucepan over medium heat, combine apple juice, remaining cinnamon, cloves, and cornstarch; bring to a boil, stirring constantly until thickened.

4 Place apples in a large bowl. Pour thickened mixture over apples and stir until evenly coated. Place apple mixture into prepared pie plate. Sprinkle crumb mixture evenly over top, gently packing it down.

5 Bake 50 to 60 minutes, or until topping is golden. Let cool, and serve.

Choices/Exchanges, 1 1/2 carbohydrate

Calories 120, Calories From Fat 15, **Total Fat** 1.5g, Saturated Fat 0.0g, Trans Fat 0.0g, **Cholesterol** 0mg, **Sodium** 10mg, **Potassium** 140mg, **Total Carbohydrates** 26g, Fiber 3g, Sugar 16g, **Protein** 1g, **Phosphorus** 40mg

Diner-Style Chocolate Cream Pie

Serves 12, 1 slice per serving

5	low-fat graham cracker sheets, finely crushed
4	tablespoons (1/4 cup) light, trans-fat-free margarine
1	tablespoon plus 1/2 cup sugar, divided
1/4	cup unsweetened cocoa powder
3	tablespoons cornstarch
1/4	teaspoon salt
2-1/4	cups fat-free milk
1	teaspoon vanilla extract
1	(8-ounce) package fat-free frozen whipped topping, thawed

1 For pie crust, in a bowl, combine graham crackers, margarine, and 1 tablespoon sugar. Press into bottom and sides of a 9-inch pie plate. Refrigerate until ready to fill.

2 In a saucepan, combine remaining sugar, cocoa, cornstarch, and salt. Gradually stir in milk. Bring to a boil over medium heat, stirring constantly.

3 Remove from heat and stir in vanilla. Pour into pie crust and chill 1 hour.

4 Spread whipped topping evenly over pie; cover loosely, and chill at least 6 hours, or until set. Cut into 12 slices and serve.

Serving Suggestion
To fancy this up, you can always sprinkle the top with a few mini chocolate chips or some shaved chocolate. Just make sure you don't overdo it.

Choices/Exchanges, 2 carbohydrate

Calories 130, Calories From Fat 20, **Total Fat** 2.0g, Saturated Fat 0.0g, Trans Fat 0.0g, **Cholesterol** 0mg, **Sodium** 200mg, **Potassium** 130mg, **Total Carbohydrates** 26g, Fiber 1g, Sugar 12g, **Protein** 3g, **Phosphorus** 60mg

Crustless Southern Pumpkin Pie

Serves 8, 1 slice per serving

1	cup fat-free evaporated milk (from a 12-ounce can)
1	cup canned pumpkin (not pumpkin pie mix)
1/2	cup granulated Splenda
1/2	cup pancake & baking mix
1	tablespoon light, trans-fat-free margarine, softened
1	teaspoon vanilla extract
1	teaspoon cinnamon, divided
1/2	teaspoon ground ginger
1/8	teaspoon allspice
1/8	teaspoon nutmeg
2	eggs
1/2	cup chopped pecans
1-1/2	cups frozen fat-free whipped topping, thawed

1 Preheat oven to 350°F. Coat a 9-inch pie plate with cooking spray.

2 In a medium bowl, combine milk, pumpkin, Splenda, baking mix, margarine, vanilla, 3/4 teaspoon cinnamon, ginger, allspice, nutmeg, and eggs until well blended. Stir in chopped pecans. Pour into pie plate.

3 Bake 35 to 40 minutes, or until knife inserted in center comes out clean. Cool completely, about 1 hour.

4 In a small bowl, stir together whipped topping and remaining cinnamon; garnish pie with topping. Cut into 8 slices and serve.

Serving Suggestion

Sometimes little extras can look so nice ... add a pecan half to each slice for that extra-special touch.

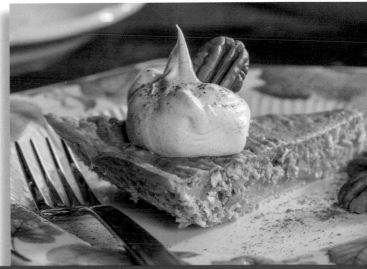

Choices/Exchanges, 1 carbohydrate, 2 fat

Calories 160, Calories From Fat 80, **Total Fat** 9.0g, Saturated Fat 1.5g, Trans Fat 0.0g, **Cholesterol** 55mg, **Sodium** 150mg, **Potassium** 240mg, **Total Carbohydrates** 15g, Fiber 2g, Sugar 6g, **Protein** 6g, **Phosphorus** 165mg

Chocolate Chip Cheesecake Cupcakes

Serves 18, 1 cupcake per serving

4	ounces fat-free cream cheese, softened
1-1/3	cups sugar, divided
1/4	cup liquid egg substitute
1/3	cup semisweet chocolate chips
1-1/2	cups all-purpose flour
1/4	cup unsweetened cocoa powder
1/4	teaspoon baking soda
1	teaspoon baking powder
1/8	teaspoon salt
1	cup water
1/3	cup canola oil
1	teaspoon vanilla extract
1	tablespoon white vinegar

1 Preheat oven to 350°F. Line 18 muffin cups with paper liners; set aside.

2 In a medium bowl, with an electric mixer on medium speed, beat cream cheese and 1/3 cup sugar for 1 minute, or until light and fluffy. Add liquid egg and beat for 1 minute, or until smooth. Stir in chocolate chips; set aside.

3 In a large bowl, combine flour, remaining sugar, cocoa powder, baking soda, baking powder, and salt. Add water, oil, vanilla, and vinegar. Beat with electric mixer on medium speed for 2 minutes, scraping down sides of bowl occasionally.

4 Spoon batter into prepared muffin cups, filling each about 1/2 full. Spoon about 1 tablespoon cream cheese mixture over each.

5 Bake 25 to 30 minutes, or until toothpick inserted in center comes out clean. Cool on wire rack 10 minutes, then remove from muffin cups and cool completely.

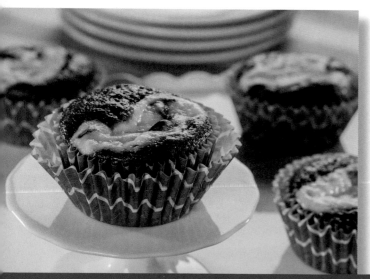

Choices/Exchanges, 2 carbohydrate, 1/2 fat

Calories 160, Calories From Fat 45, **Total Fat** 5.0g, Saturated Fat 1.0g, Trans Fat 0.0g, **Cholesterol** 0mg, **Sodium** 100mg, **Potassium** 55mg, **Total Carbohydrates** 26g, Fiber <1g, Sugar 15g, **Protein** 3g, **Phosphorus** 55mg

Sandwich Cookie Cupcakes

Serves 24, 1 cupcake per serving

1	(18.25-ounce) package white cake mix
1-1/4	cups water
1/4	cup canola oil
3	egg whites
1	cup coarsely crushed sugar-free chocolate sandwich cookies, divided
3/4	(12-ounce) container sugar-free vanilla frosting

1 Preheat oven to 350°F. Line 24 muffin cups with paper liners.

2 In a large bowl, with an electric mixer on low speed, beat cake mix, water, oil, and egg whites 30 seconds, then beat on high 2 minutes. Gently fold in 3/4 cup crushed cookies.

3 Spoon batter into muffin cups, filling each about 2/3 full.

4 Bake 18 to 22 minutes, or until a toothpick inserted in center comes out clean. Cool completely, then frost. Sprinkle with remaining crushed cookies.

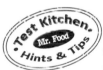

To crush the sandwich cookies, simply put them in a plastic bag and gently tap or roll over them with a rolling pin or soup can. Not only does this work perfectly, it's also a great stress reliever.

Choices/Exchanges, 2 carbohydrate, 1 fat

Calories 160, Calories From Fat 60, **Total Fat** 7.0g, Saturated Fat 1.5g, Trans Fat 0.5g, **Cholesterol** 0mg, **Sodium** 170mg, **Potassium** 20mg, **Total Carbohydrates** 27g, Fiber 1g, Sugar 0g, **Protein** 2g, **Phosphorus** 70mg

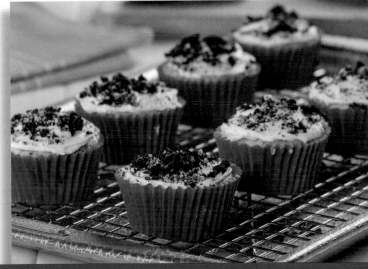

Strawberry Shortcake Roll

Serves 12, 1 slice per serving

4	eggs, separated
3/4	cup granulated sugar
1	tablespoon plus 1 teaspoon vanilla extract, divided
3/4	cup all-purpose flour
3/4	teaspoon baking powder
1/4	teaspoon salt
2	tablespoons confectioners' sugar, divided, plus extra for sprinkling
1	(8-ounce) package fat-free cream cheese, softened
1	(8-ounce) container frozen reduced-fat whipped topping, thawed
1	cup finely chopped strawberries

1 Preheat oven to 400°F. Line a 10 × 15-inch jelly roll pan with wax paper.

2 In a medium bowl, with an electric mixer, beat egg whites until stiff peaks form; set aside. In a large bowl, beat egg yolks until light. Gradually add the granulated sugar and 1 tablespoon vanilla, and mix well.

3 In a third bowl, sift together the flour, baking powder, and salt, and add to the egg yolk mixture. Fold the egg whites into the egg yolk mixture and pour batter into prepared pan.

4 Bake 7 to 9 minutes, or until cake is golden. Loosen edges of cake and turn cake onto kitchen towel dusted with 1 tablespoon confectioners' sugar. Gently peel off wax paper. Roll up jelly roll-style in the towel, starting with a short side. Cool on a wire rack.

5 In a large bowl, beat together cream cheese, remaining vanilla, and remaining confectioners' sugar. Fold in the whipped topping, then fold in strawberries. Unroll cake and spread filling evenly over cake to within 1/2 inch of edges; roll up. Cover and refrigerate until ready to serve. Sprinkle with a little extra confectioners' sugar, cut into 12 slices, and serve.

Test Kitchen Mr. Food Hints & Tips

The reason we roll the cake up in a towel while it's still warm is so that it won't crack when you re-roll it after it cools. And ya can't fill it while it's warm or the filling will melt. See, it all makes sense now.

Choices/Exchanges, 1 1/2 carbohydrate, 1/2 fat

Calories 130, Calories From Fat 20, **Total Fat** 2.0g, Saturated Fat 0.5g, Trans Fat 0.0g, **Cholesterol** 70mg, **Sodium** 210mg, **Potassium** 85mg, **Total Carbohydrates** 22g, Fiber 0g, Sugar 14g, **Protein** 6g, **Phosphorus** 130mg

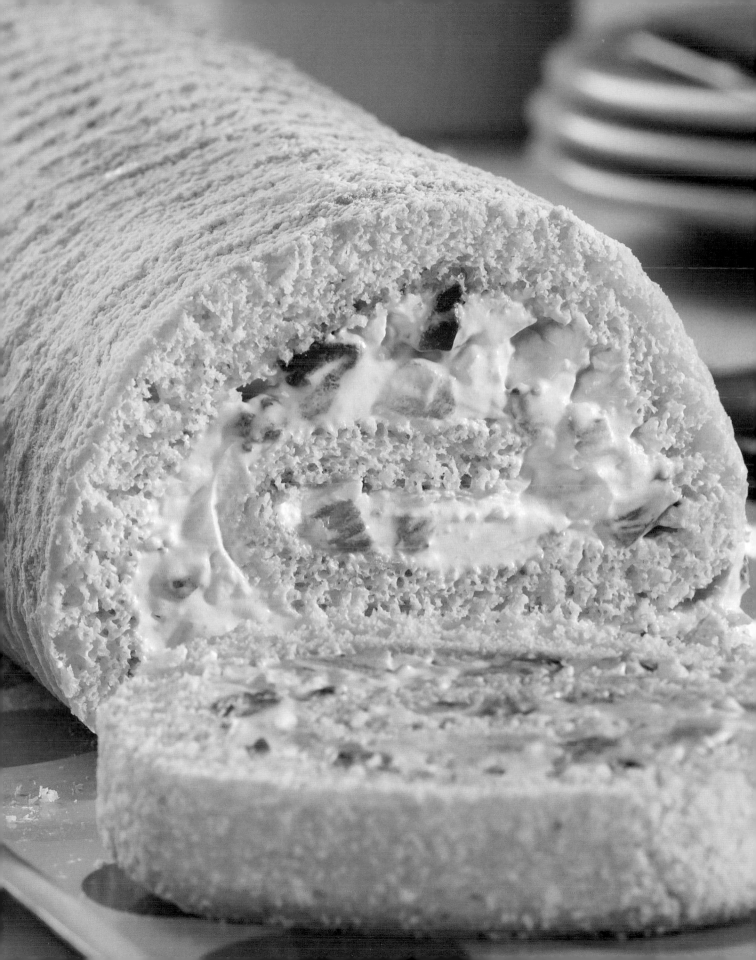

Very Berry Tart

Serves 6, 1/6 tart per serving

2	eggs
1/4	cup sugar
1	teaspoon vanilla extract
1/8	teaspoon salt
1	cup fat-free milk
1/2	cup all-purpose flour
1/2	teaspoon baking powder
3	cups assorted fresh berries (such as raspberries, blueberries, and/or sliced strawberries)

1 Preheat oven to 400°F. Lightly coat a 9-inch deep dish pie plate or quiche pan with cooking spray.

2 In a medium bowl, combine eggs, sugar, vanilla, and salt; whisk until light and frothy. Whisk in milk until combined. Add flour and baking powder; whisk until smooth.

3 Place berries in prepared pie plate; pour batter over berries. (Batter will not cover berries completely.)

4 Bake about 20 minutes, or until puffed and golden brown. Cut into 6 slices and serve warm.

Did You Know?
This is a very moist tart, sort of a cross between a flan and a Dutch pancake. That means it would be as welcome at breakfast as it would with a cup of coffee for dessert.

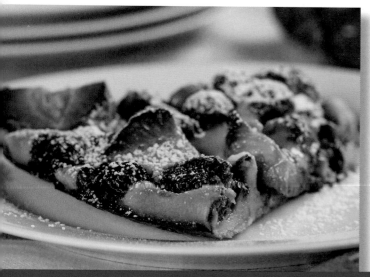

Choices/Exchanges, 2 carbohydrate

Calories 150, Calories From Fat 20, **Total Fat** 2.0g, Saturated Fat 0.5g, Trans Fat 0.0g, **Cholesterol** 65mg, **Sodium** 120mg, **Potassium** 190mg, **Total Carbohydrates** 27g, Fiber 3g, Sugar 15g, **Protein** 5g, **Phosphorus** 140mg

Minty Watermelon Ice

Serves 10, 3/4 cup per serving

3/4	cup water
1/3	cup granulated Splenda
5	cups seeded watermelon cubes
1/3	cup fresh mint
2	tablespoons lime juice

1 In a small bowl, combine water and Splenda, stirring until dissolved.

2 In a blender or food processor, combine watermelon, mint, and lime juice, blending until nearly smooth. Add Splenda mixture; blend until smooth.

3 Transfer to a 9 × 13-inch baking dish. Cover and freeze about 2-1/2 hours, or until almost solid.

4 Using a fork, scrape the mixture into shaved crystals. Spoon into individual dishes and serve immediately, or cover and refreeze until ready to serve.

Did You Know?
You can call this an ice, slush, or even a granita; it's up to you. All we know for sure is that we call it amazingly refreshing.

Choices/Exchanges, 1/2 carbohydrate

Calories 25, Calories From Fat 0, **Total Fat** 0.0g, Saturated Fat 0.0g, Trans Fat 0.0g, **Cholesterol** 0mg, **Sodium** 0mg, **Potassium** 95mg, **Total Carbohydrates** 6g, Fiber 0g, Sugar 5g, **Protein** <1g, **Phosphorus** 10mg

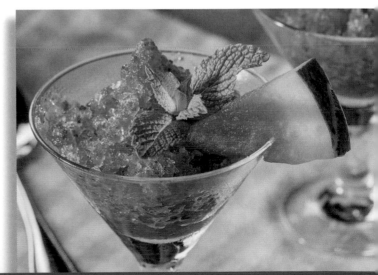

Heavenly Banana Pudding

Serves 10, about 1 cup per serving

2   (4-serving-size) packages sugar-free instant white chocolate pudding mix

4   cups fat-free milk

20   reduced-fat vanilla wafers, coarsely crushed

4   cups sliced bananas

1   (8-ounce) container reduced-fat frozen whipped topping, thawed

1 In a medium bowl, combine pudding mix and milk; mix well.

2 In a large glass bowl, spread half the pudding, half the wafer crumbs, half the banana slices, then half the whipped topping. Repeat layers. Serve immediately, or chill until ready to serve.

Serving Suggestion

How about serving this in individual parfait glasses? Just layer even amounts of ingredients into each glass for a dessert that not only looks fancy, but tastes great, too!

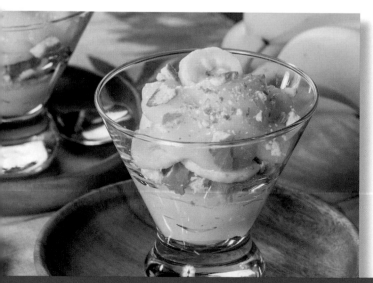

Choices/Exchanges, 2 carbohydrate

Calories 140, Calories From Fat 15, **Total Fat** 1.5g, Saturated Fat 0.0g, Trans Fat 0.0g, **Cholesterol** 5mg, **Sodium** 290mg, **Potassium** 380mg, **Total Carbohydrates** 28g, Fiber 2g, Sugar 14g, **Protein** 4g, **Phosphorus** 120mg

Mixed Berry Freeze

Serves 6, about 3/4 cup per serving

1	(16-ounce) package frozen mixed berries, slightly thawed
1	(8-ounce) cup low-fat vanilla Greek yogurt
6	tablespoons granulated Splenda
2	tablespoons honey
1/2	teaspoon vanilla extract

1 Place berries into a food processor. Process until fruit is chopped into small pieces.

2 Add yogurt, Splenda, honey, and vanilla, and process until smooth, scraping down sides as needed.

3 Serve immediately for a softer consistency, or spoon into a container, cover, and freeze 4 to 6 hours, or until firm.

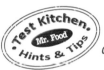

For extra-creamy yogurt, once the mixture has frozen, break it up and process it again in a food processor before serving.

Choices/Exchanges, 1 carbohydrate

Calories 90, Calories From Fat 10, **Total Fat** 1.0g, Saturated Fat 0.0g, Trans Fat 0.0g, **Cholesterol** <5mg, **Sodium** 15mg, **Potassium** 90mg, **Total Carbohydrates** 16g, Fiber 2g, Sugar 13g, **Protein** 4g, **Phosphorus** 15mg

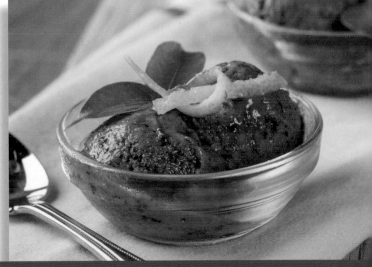

Patchwork Quilt Loaf

Serves 10, 1 slice per serving

1   (4-serving-size) package sugar-free strawberry-flavored gelatin

1   (4-serving-size) package sugar-free orange-flavored gelatin

1   (4-serving-size) package sugar-free lime-flavored gelatin

4   cups boiling water, divided

1-1/4   cups cold water, divided

1   (4-serving-size) package sugar-free lemon-flavored gelatin

1/4   cup sugar

1   (8-ounce) container frozen fat-free whipped topping, thawed

1 Coat 3 (2-cup) square plastic containers with cooking spray.

2 Prepare the strawberry, orange, and lime gelatins separately by dissolving each in 1 cup boiling water; stir until completely dissolved. Add 1/4 cup cold water to each, then pour each into a separate container.

3 Chill about 1-1/2 hours or until firm, then cut each gelatin into 1-inch cubes. Cover and set aside in the refrigerator.

4 In a large bowl, dissolve lemon gelatin and sugar in remaining boiling water and stir in remaining cold water. Chill until slightly thickened, about 30 minutes. Fold in whipped topping; mix well. Fold in gelatin cubes and pour into a 9 × 5-inch loaf pan that has been coated with cooking spray. Refrigerate 8 hours or overnight.

5 When ready to serve, run a knife around edge. Gently shake pan to loosen the dessert; invert onto a serving platter. Cut into 10 slices and serve immediately.

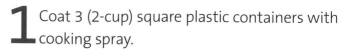

Use gelatin colors/flavors that are seasonal for a festive look! Red and green at Christmas, orange and yellow for Thanksgiving. You get the idea.

Choices/Exchanges, 1/2 carbohydrate

Calories 30, Calories From Fat 0, **Total Fat** 0.0g, Saturated Fat 0.0g, Trans Fat 0.0g, **Cholesterol** 0mg, **Sodium** 70mg, **Potassium** 0mg, **Total Carbohydrates** 6g, Fiber 0g, Sugar 5g, **Protein** 2g, **Phosphorus** 40mg

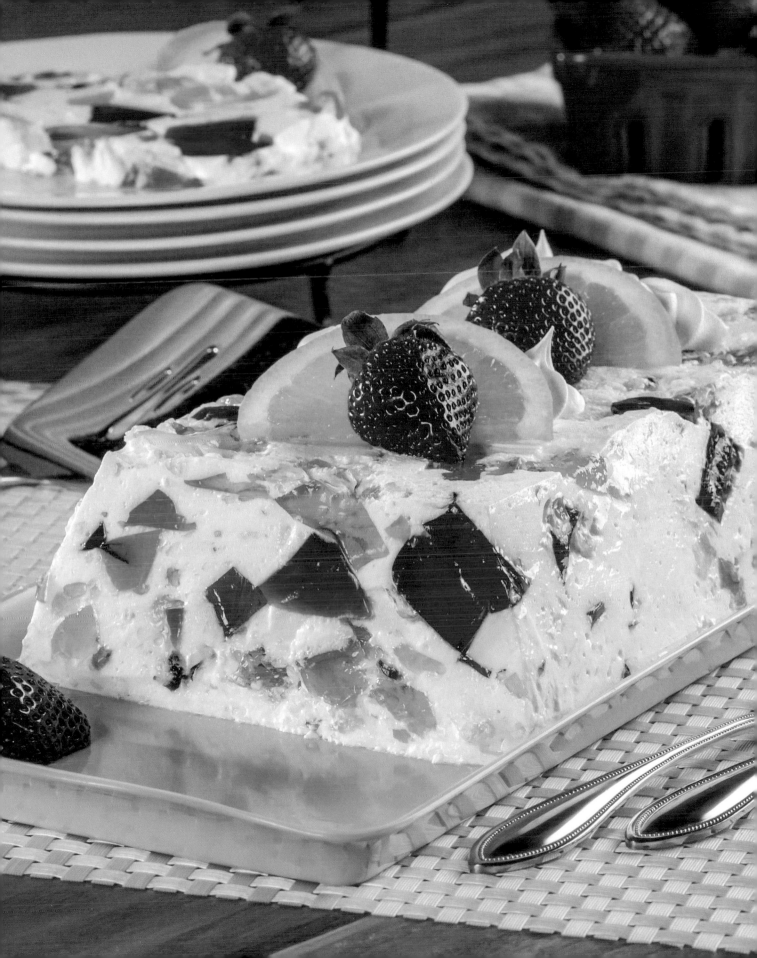

Super Easy Nut Clusters

Serves 28, 1 cluster per serving

1 cup sugar-free chocolate chips
1 cup coarsely chopped mixed nuts, plus 1/3 cup extra for garnish, if desired

1 Line 28 mini muffin cups with paper liners.

2 Place chocolate chips in a microwaveable bowl; microwave until almost melted, stirring every 30 seconds to prevent overheating them. Remove from microwave when chocolate is mostly melted, and continue stirring until chocolate is entirely melted and smooth.

3 Add 1 cup nuts to melted chocolate and stir until well mixed and all pieces are coated.

4 Using a teaspoon, evenly drop small spoonfuls of mixture into prepared muffin cups. Garnish with a sprinkle of chopped nuts, if desired, before chocolate sets.

5 Place clusters in refrigerator for 20 minutes before serving, to set chocolate completely.

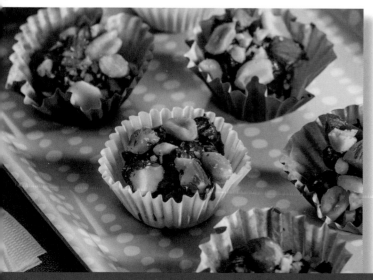

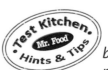

Since you probably have both ingredients for this in your pantry, it's a great treat to throw together when last-minute company is on the way.

Test Kitchen Mr. Food Hints & Tips

Choices/Exchanges, 1/2 carbohydrate, 1 fat

Calories 60, Calories From Fat 40, **Total Fat** 4.5g, Saturated Fat 1.5g, Trans Fat 0.0g, **Cholesterol** 0mg, **Sodium** 0mg, **Potassium** 35mg, **Total Carbohydrates** 5g, Fiber 0g, Sugar 0g, **Protein** 1g, **Phosphorus** 20mg

"Puppy Chow" Snack Mix

Serves 8, about 1/4 cup per serving

2	cups honey squares cereal with fiber (we tested these with Fiber One Honey Squares)
2	tablespoons light, trans-fat-free margarine
2	tablespoons creamy peanut butter
1/4	cup sugar-free chocolate chips
1	(4-serving-size) package sugar-free vanilla pudding mix

1 Place cereal in a large bowl; set aside.

2 In a small saucepan over low heat, combine margarine, peanut butter, and chocolate chips, stirring constantly until melted. Mix well and pour over cereal; stir to coat evenly. Let cool about 20 minutes.

3 Once mixture has cooled, pour into a large, resealable plastic bag. Add pudding mix and shake gently to coat evenly. Store in an airtight container.

Did You Know?

We named this "Puppy Chow" only because it looks like it. It's not intended to serve to dogs. Of course you know that, since chocolate is always considered off-limits to man's best friend.

Choices/Exchanges, 1 carbohydrate, 1/2 fat

Calories 90, Calories From Fat 45, **Total Fat** 5.0g, Saturated Fat 1.5g, Trans Fat 0.0g, **Cholesterol** 0mg, **Sodium** 240mg, **Potassium** 50mg, **Total Carbohydrates** 15g, Fiber 4g, Sugar 1g, **Protein** 1g, **Phosphorus** 100mg

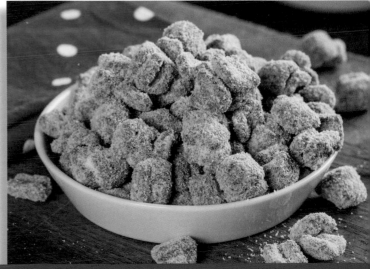

Index